Overview of Target-Controlled Infusions
and Total Intravenous Anaesthesia

Overview of Target-Controlled Infusions and Total Intravenous Anaesthesia

Third Edition

Anthony R Absalom

Professor of Anesthesiology

Dept. of Anesthesiology, University Medical Center Groningen, Groningen University

Groningen, The Netherlands

Michel MRF Struys

Professor and Chair, Dept. of Anesthesiology, University Medical Center Groningen

Groningen University, Groningen, The Netherlands

and

Professor, Dept. of Basic and Applied Medical Sciences, Ghent University, Gent, Belgium

ACADEMIA
PRESS

Acknowledgements: The authors are grateful to the following for their assistance during the preparation of this book: Kai van Amsterdam, MSc, Douglas Eleveld, PhD and Mendy Driesens, PA (department of Anesthesiology, UMCG, Groningen); and Tom De Smet, PhD (Demed Medical, Temse, Belgium).

Academia Press
Ampla House
Coupure Rechts 88
9000 Gent
België

www.academiapress.be

Academia Press is a subsidiary of Lannoo Publishers.

2nd printing, 2020

ISBN 9789401462839
D/2019/45/374
NUR 876

Anthony Absalom & Michel MRF Struys
An Overview of TCI & TIVA
Gent, Academia Press, 2019, 112 p.

Cover: Cheryl Keates
Layout: Crius Group

Contents

General and historical background

Total intravenous anaesthesia (TIVA) – when anaesthesia is induced and maintained with intravenous anaesthetic drugs – has been a relatively recent addition to the anaesthetists' repertoire. Although intravenous induction of anaesthesia became common in the 1930's after the discovery of the barbiturates, intravenous maintenance of anaesthesia only became practical, safe and popular after the introduction of propofol into clinical practice in the 1990s. First used clinically in 1977, propofol is the only currently available intravenous hypnotic agent suitable for induction and maintenance of anaesthesia. The discovery, in recent decades, of the shorter-acting opioid analgesics alfentanil and remifentanil, which have a rapid onset and offset of action and are eminently suitable for use by infusion, coupled with technological developments (such as more reliable and accurate intravenous pumps), and advances in our understanding of pharmacokinetic principles have enabled the development of the technique of TIVA in which anaesthesia is administered exclusively via the intravenous route.

Propofol-based TIVA techniques have many advantages. These include rapid recovery of consciousness and psychomotor function, earlier recovery and discharge from the post-anaesthesia care unit and shorter times to achieve 'home-readiness' than inhalational anaesthetic techniques.[1 2] Propofol has an anti-emetic affect,[3] and is thus associated with a lower incidence of postoperative nausea and vomiting.[4-9] Intravenous agents have no known adverse effects on theatre staff. Whereas exhaled inhalational agents contribute directly and significantly to the greenhouse gases, the greenhouse gas emissions arising from propofol use are miniscule (four orders of magnitude less than N_2O and desflurane) as they only arise during manufacture, transport, and the syringe pump operation.[10] It should however be mentioned that unused propofol should always be incinerated with clinical waste. If discarded into the water drains it is toxic to the aquatic environment.[11]

Significant advances during the past decades in our understanding of the pharmacokinetics and pharmacodynamics of the anaesthetic drugs has generated the knowledge required for rational administration of these drugs. The ultimate goal, when administering a particular dose of drug, is a specified clinical effect, for which a specific therapeutic concentration at the site of drug action is

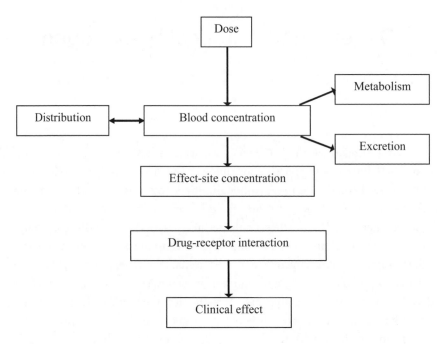

Figure 1: Schematic representation of the pharmacokinetic and dynamic processes determining the relationship between administered dose and resulting clinical effect.

necessary. This dose-response relationship, summarised in Figure 1, can be divided into three parts: the relationship between dose administered and plasma concentration (the pharmacokinetic phase), the relationship between effect organ concentration and clinical effect (the pharmacodynamic phase) and the coupling between pharmacokinetics and dynamics.

For several decades anaesthetists have been able to titrate the blood concentration of the inhalational anaesthetic agents by using a vapouriser to administer the drug and by measuring the end-tidal concentration (a moderately accurate estimate of blood concentration). In this way, anaesthetists who use inhalational anaesthesia need mainly to concern themselves with the pharmacodynamic phase of the dose response relationship.

The introduction of target-controlled infusion (TCI) technology in the late 1990s provided a similar facility to administer stable predicted plasma concentrations of the intravenous anaesthetic agents. Before this anaesthetists administering intravenous anaesthetic agents tended to calculate the dose or infusion rate according to the weight of the patient. The problem with this is the complex relationship between dose, plasma and effect-site concentrations. Simple infusion regimens do not yield steady state plasma concentration profiles until at least 5 multiples of the elimination half-life. Also, the calculations required to estimate the plasma and effect-site concentrations are complex and not amenable to mental arithmetic! While encouraging progress has been made with methods of online estimation of blood propofol concentrations from measurement of exhaled gas concentrations of propofol metabolites, [12-16] and with point of care plasma propofol measurements,[17] these systems, even though since recently commercially available, require further refinement and development before they can become a useful pharmacological addition to the anaesthetists' clinical decision tools.

1
—

Target-controlled infusions

Definition

A target-controlled infusion is an infusion where the intent is to achieve a user-defined drug concentration in a body compartment or tissue of interest. An anaesthetist using a TCI system to administer an anaesthetic agent is thus able to set a desired concentration (usually referred to as the "target concentration"), and to change the target concentration based on the observed responses to the set target concentration. TCI systems are programmed to use multi-compartmental pharmacokinetic models, and accompanying poly-exponential equations, to calculate the infusion rates required to achieve the target concentration (see below).

Theoretically, a TCI system can control the concentration in any compartment or tissue in the body. The pharmacokinetic models used are derived from previously performed population pharmacokinetic studies. By convention the central compartment in a pharmacokinetic model is referred to as V_c or V_1, and this compartment includes the vascular compartment. Thus when the target is a user-defined concentration in the central compartment (which includes the vascular compartment), the infusion is referred to as a plasma targeted TCI. When the target concentration is a concentration at the site of action of the drug, the infusion is referred to as an effect-site targeted TCI.

Development of TCI systems

A brief description of the history of the development of TCI systems follows (this topic was reviewed in greater detail recently[18]). In 1968 Kruger-Thiemer described a theoretical approach to maintaining and achieving a steady state plasma concentration of a drug whose pharmacokinetics can be described by a two-compartment model.[19] Vaughan and Tucker [20][21] developed the concept further, as did Schwilden who also developed the first clinical application of this theory, the CATIA system (computer-assisted total intravenous anaesthesia system).[22] The schemes developed by these pioneers for drugs whose pharmacokinetics can be described by a two-compartment model became known as BET (**B**olus, **E**limination, **T**ransfer) schemes. They were called this because they comprised an initial bolus to fill the central compartment, followed by two superimposed infusions, one to replace drug removed from the central compartment by elimination and one to replace drug that has been distributed to the peripheral compartment. A fixed proportion of the total amount of drug in the central compartment is eliminated each unit of time. Thus when the plasma concentration of a drug is constant the amount of drug eliminated each unit of time is constant, so that drug lost by elimination can be replaced by a constant rate infusion. In contrast the amount of drug distributed to peripheral tissues declines exponentially as the gradient between the central compartment and the peripheral compartment decreases. Thus an infusion at an exponentially declining rate is required to replace drug removed from the central compartment by distribution. The sum of these two infusions is naturally an infusion at a decreasing rate.

Since then it has been recognised that the pharmacokinetics of most anaesthetic agents conform best to three compartment models. Numerous algorithms, appropriate for a three compartment model, for targeting plasma concentrations [23-27] and for targeting effect-site concentrations [28][29] have been published, and several groups of investigators have developed model-driven automated systems capable of delivering steady state drug concentrations. Since the early 1990s the experimental target-controlled infusion software programs developed in Stanford (Stanpump), Stellenbosch (Stelpump), Erlangen (CATIA and IV FEED), Alabama (CACI), Leiden (Leiden TCI System), Brussels (Toolbox), Santiago (AnestFusor), and Gent (RUGLOOP) have been used to study the pharmacology of existing and new drugs and to investigate the advantages of TCI. Several other pharmacokinetic simulation programs have also been developed (see recent review [30]).

Initially different groups used different terminology to describe their systems.[22][31-34] Eventually a consensus was reached among the leading groups, who published a letter in Anesthesiology suggesting that the term TCI should be adopted.[35] The group also suggested standard nomenclature for plasma and effect-site concentrations (C_p and C_e respectively, with the added subscripts T to indicate that the concentration being discussed is the "target" concentration, CALC to indicate that the concentration is the calculated plasma or effect-site concentration, and MEAS to indicate that the plasma or effect-site concentration is a measured concentration).

The first commercially available TCI system was the Diprifusor®, a microprocessor that was embedded in intravenous infusion pumps sold by several manufacturers from 1996 onwards (in numerous countries around the world, but not in the USA). The development of the Diprifusor® has been described in detail.[18 36 37] TCI pumps controlled by it can only administer target-controlled infusions of propofol, and only if the microprocessor is able to detect the presence of single-use pre-filled glass syringes of 1 or 2% propofol purchased from AstraZeneca. These syringes contain a programmable metallic strip in the flange that is detected by a sophisticated process called programmed magnetic resonance. When the syringe is almost empty the strip is "de-programmed" so that it cannot be re-used.

A few years after the release of the first generation of TCI systems, the patent for propofol expired, resulting in significantly cheaper generic forms of propofol becoming available. This prompted the development and launch of second generation of TCI systems, the so-called "Open TCI" systems. These systems allow the use of a variety of drugs, administered from a variety of syringes and sizes. Numerous second generation systems are now available.[30]

Components of a TCI system

The basic components of a TCI system are a user interface, a computer or one or more microprocessors and an infusion device. The microprocessor controls the appearance of the user interface, implements the pharmacokinetic model, accepts data input and instructions from the user, performs the necessary mathematical calculations, controls and monitors the infusion device, and implements warning systems to alert the user of any problems (e.g. mains disconnection, syringe almost empty).

Audible and visible warning systems are an essential feature, and TCI devices should be programmed to respond appropriately to all possible fault conditions. Should a serious fault occur, then alarms should sound and the system should shut down or stop infusing, depending on the fault. The first generation TCI pumps contained two microprocessors. A 16-bit microprocessor implemented the algorithm to calculate the infusion rates required for the target concentration, and controlled the syringe driver motor speed accordingly. In parallel, an 8-bit processor monitored the number of rotations of the driving motor and used a simpler mathematical process (involving Euler approximations) to calculate the estimated plasma concentration based on the amount of propofol delivered. If the target and estimated plasma concentrations differed significantly, the system shut down. As this was a very rare occurrence and faster microprocessors had been developed, the dual processor technique has not been implemented in the new generation pumps.

The user interface prompts and allows the user to enter the patient data such as age, weight, gender and height and of course the target drug concentration, whilst displaying useful numeric and/or graphic information (such as the current infusion rate, and the trend of the calculated plasma and effect-site drug concentrations). Typical TCI systems incorporate infusion devices that are capable of infusion rates up to 1200 ml/hr, with a precision of at least 0.1 ml/hr.

Plasma concentration targeted TCI

HOW DO PLASMA-TARGETED TCI SYSTEMS DELIVER STEADY STATE PLASMA CONCENTRATIONS?

TCI systems are programmed with pharmacokinetic models that mathematically describe the processes of drug distribution and elimination (see Figure 2 and also the later section on pharmacokinetic models). Although different TCI systems might use slightly different mathematical techniques, the practical end result remains a variation of a BET scheme.

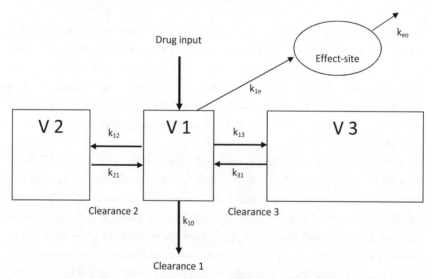

Figure 2: The three compartment pharmacokinetic model enlarged with an effect compartment. The concentration in this compartment is called "effect-site concentration".

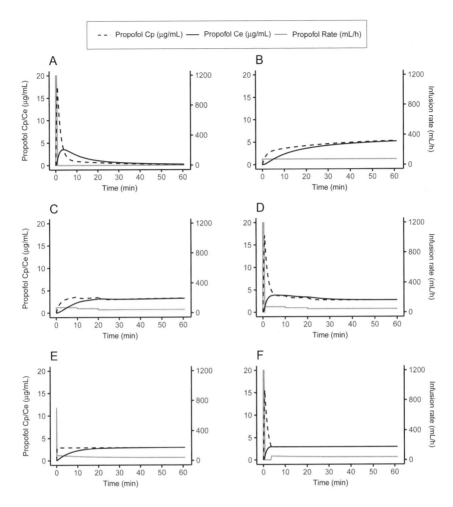

Figure 3: Propofol plasma and effect-site concentrations of various propofol infusion schemes predicted by the Eleveld model. A: bolus 2 mg/mg at 1200 ml/h; B: continuous infusion at 10 mg/kg/h; C: Continuous infusion of 10 – 8 – 6 mg/kg/h (10 minute intervals between decrements) ; D: bolus 2 mg/kg, followed by a 10 – 8 – 6 mg/kg/h continuous infusion (10 minute intervals between decrements) ; E: plasma targeted TCI at 2.89 µg/ml ; effect-site targeted TCI at 2.89 µg/ml. Patient is male, 170 cm, 75 kg, 45 years.

The general method is illustrated in Figure 3. When the anaesthetist increases the target concentration the system administers a rapid infusion (bolus) to quickly fill the central compartment thereby giving an almost step-wise increase in plasma concentration. The amount infused is calculated according to the estimated central compartment plasma volume and the difference between the current calculated concentration and the target concentrations. When the system calculates that the plasma concentration has reached its new target, it stops the rapid infusion, and commences an infusion at a lower rate. For practical reasons, current TCI systems repeat the calculations, and alter the infusion rate, at discrete intervals (typically every 10 sec). Thus, although the amount of drug removed from the central compartment changes continuously, the infusion rate changes in a "step-wise decreasing" manner. If a three compartment model is in use, three superimposed infusions are required. While the target concentration is constant, a constant rate infusion is required to replace drug removed by elimination. Two first-order infusions – at exponentially decreasing infusion rates – are required to match the net movement of drug from the central to the other two compartments. The net result is a slowly decreasing infusion rate over time (until total steady-state is reached, which requires an infusion lasting > 24 hours). This is shown in figure 3, panel E.

When the anaesthetist decreases the target concentration the system stops the infusion, and waits until it estimates that the plasma concentration has reached the target concentration. The rate at which the plasma concentration falls depends on the rate of elimination, and on the gradient between the concentrations in the central and other compartments. Thus if the concentration in the central compartment is greater than that in another compartment, the plasma concentration will fall more rapidly, whereas if the reverse is true, the return of drug from the peripheral compartment will reduce the rate of decline in the plasma concentration. Once the system estimates the plasma concentration has reached the target, it will re-start the infusion at a lower rate, once again calculating the changing infusion rates required to maintain the plasma concentration at the target concentration.

TCI VS MANUAL INFUSIONS

Although pharmacological models exists for all drugs, in most areas of medical practice doctors tend to use manually controlled infusions, usually at a fixed rate. Target-controlled infusion systems automatically take into account drug accumulation over time (without the user having to adapt the infusion rate manually) and this gives the clinician more precise control of plasma and effect-site concentrations. Certainly in anaesthesia, where it is important for the clinician to be able to exert fine, rapid control over specific drug concentrations, TCI offers benefits.

With most drugs administered by a fixed rate infusion, the plasma concentrations take a long time to reach a plateau or steady state. This is illustrated for propofol in Figure 3, panel B, which shows that after 60 minutes, the plasma concentration is still rising. In fact, plasma concentrations will continue rising for >12 hours, since it takes >24 hours for the drug to equilibrate throughout all the tissues in the body. For drugs such as fentanyl, morphine and midazolam, the time taken for equilibration and steady state is even longer.

For the latter drugs and also for propofol large changes to an infusion rate will not lead to significant changes in plasma concentration for some time (see Figure 3, panel C – at 10 minutes the infusion rate from 10 to 8 mg/kg/hr, and after another 10 minutes to 6 mg/kg/hr, but despite these sizeable changes, the plasma propofol concentration undergoes a proportionally far smaller change. The time delay before there is a significant change in effect-site concentration, and thus in clinical effect, will be even longer.

When a rapid increase in the drug concentration is needed then this is best achieved by administration of a bolus, but it is difficult to judge the size of bolus appropriate for the patient and the desired change in plasma or effect-site concentration (see Figure 3, panel D). Similarly, to decrease the concentration as rapidly as possible, it is best to switch off the infusion temporarily, but in the busy theatre environment there is a real risk the anaesthetist may forget to re-start the infusion. With TCI systems, these changes are made automatically, enabling precise and rapid control of the plasma concentration.

It is not surprising that TCI systems are popular with anaesthetists, who have assessed them as easy to use, and providing a high level of predictability of anaesthetic effect.[38] In a study comparing manual infusion with TCI propofol by anaesthetists unfamiliar with propofol infusion anaesthesia, it was found that anaesthetists quickly became familiar with both techniques, but expressed a clear preference for the TCI system.[39] A multicentre study found that the control of anaesthesia was easier in subjects anaesthetised with target-controlled than with manually controlled propofol infusions.[40]

How does the quality of clinical control compare between TCI and manually controlled infusions? Although many of the early target-controlled infusion systems were used for infusions of opiates, most of the evidence comes from studies comparing TCI with manually controlled propofol infusions. Quality of anaesthesia is difficult to measure, but studies have used simple categorical measures where the anaesthetist rates the quality as good, adequate or poor as well as other numerical methods such as a quality of anaesthesia score. [41] In studies comparing TCI with manual propofol infusion regimens the quality of induction and maintenance of anaesthesia the incidence and severity of haemodynamic effects, and the recovery times were either similar or better with TCI administration.[39] [42-47] Despite this, there is no strong evidence that TCI administration is associated with better outcomes than manual administration.[48]

Effect-site concentration targeted TCI

The first generation TCI systems incorporated the Diprifusor microprocessor which is programmed to target the plasma concentration. Although some systems displayed the estimated effect-site concentration, they did not allow effect-site targeting. The disadvantage of targeting the plasma concentration is that when the target concentration is changed there is a temporal delay before the plasma and effect-site concentrations equilibrate. This is clearly illustrated in Figure 3 panel E. As the clinical effect of a drug depends on the concentration at the effect-site, there is an hysteresis in clinical effect when the target plasma concentration of the agent is increased or decreased. In fact it was, in part, the observation made by anaesthetists using early propofol TCI systems that patients lost and regained consciousness at different estimated plasma concentrations that lead to the realisation that plasma-effect-site equilibration is not instantaneous; and that when plasma concentrations were changing it was the effect-site and not the plasma concentration that determined the clinical effect.

The rate of equilibration between plasma and effect-site depends on several factors. These include the factors that influence the rate of delivery of the drug to the effect-site (such as cardiac output and cerebral blood flow), the plasma-effect-site concentration gradient, and the pharmacological properties of the drug that determine the rate of transfer of the drug across the blood-brain barrier (lipid solubility, degree of ionisation etc). The time course of plasma-effect-site equilibration can be mathematically described by a rate constant typically referred to as the k_{eo}. Strictly speaking k_{eo} should be used to describe the rate of removal of drug from the effect-site out of the body, but the effect-site is usually regarded as a volume-less additional compartment, so that there is no need for separate constants describing the rate constants for movement into *and out of* the effect compartment.

Naturally the concentration at the effect-site cannot be directly measured, and most of the time the plasma concentration is not known either. However, the time-course of the changes in the effect-site concentration can be estimated from measures of clinical effect such as spontaneous or evoked EEG parameters. When plasma concentrations and clinical effect are measured concurrently, the k_{eo} can be estimated using mathematical modelling [49] [50] and incorporated in a combined pharmacokinetic-pharmacodynamic model may be applicable to a similar population.

When pharmacokinetic and pharmacodynamic data are not available from the same subject group then it is recommended that the time to peak effect (TTPE), a model-independent parameter, is used to estimate the k_{eo} for a

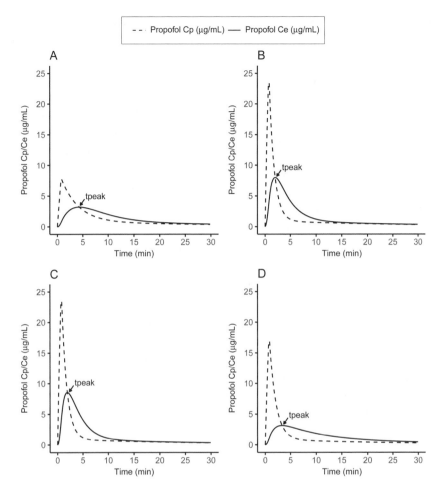

Figure 4: Predicted plasma and effect-site concentration of a propofol (10 mg/ml) bolus 2 mg/kg using the Marsh model (A), Schnider model with fixed ke0 (B), Schnider model using fixed tpeak (C), and the Eleveld model (D). The tpeak is indicated for every model. Patient is male, 170 cm, 75 kg, 45 years.

pharmacokinetic model and patient group.[51] For a given patient, and a given drug, bolus administration of a drug will result in a rapid increase in plasma concentration, followed by a bi- or tri-exponential decline, the rate of which is determined by the pharmacokinetic characteristics of the drug. When the plasma concentration is greater than the concentration in the effect-site, the effect-site concentration rises, and vice versa. After a bolus the maximum effect-site drug concentration occurs at the point when the plasma and effect-site concentration curves cross (see Figure 4). As the clinical effect is determined by the effect-site concentration, the time delay between a bolus injection and the time at which the plasma and effect-site concentration curves cross or intersect, is referred to as the "time to peak effect" (TTPE). It is important to remember that in general, the time to peak effect of a given drug in a given patient is independent of the size of the bolus dose.

After a standard bolus dose calculated on a mg/kg basis, a simple model such as the Marsh model,[52] in which all volumes and clearances scale linearly with weight, will predict the same peak plasma concentration, and the same time-course of plasma drug concentration, for all patients, regardless of their age, weight, gender or height. In this case, the same TTPE will generate the same k_{eo} for all patients. More complex multivariate models also include height, weight and gender as co-variates (e.g. Schnider,[53 54] Minto[55 56] or Eleveld[57]). For the same dose calculated on a mg/kg basis, complex models will predict different peaks and/or time-courses of plasma concentrations for patients with different gender, height or weight. In this case, if the TTPE for that drug and population is known, then that TTPE can be used to calculate a unique k_{eo} for each patient.[58]

When a combined pharmacokinetic-dynamic model is available it is possible to "target" the effect-site rather than the plasma concentration. With effect-site targeting the system manipulates the plasma concentration to bring about the target (effect-site) concentration as rapidly as possible without an overshoot of the effect-site concentration. This is illustrated in Figure 3, panel F. A more detailed example is shown in Figure 5.

When the target effect-site concentration is increased the system calculates an optimal peak plasma concentration that will cause a gradient sufficient to cause the most rapid increase in effect-site concentration but without an overshoot of the effect-site concentration. Once the system estimates that this calculated plasma concentration has been reached the infusion is switched off. If the peak was calculated correctly the (declining) plasma and (increasing) effect-site concentrations will reach the target simultaneously. The system will then restart the infusion to maintain the plasma (and effect-site) concentrations at the target concentration.

If the target effect-site concentration is decreased the system switches off the infusion, and allows the plasma concentration to fall below the target level, thereby creating a gradient driving drug out of the effect-site. This causes the most rapid possible decline in effect-site concentration. As soon as the effect-site concentration reaches the target, the infusion is re-started. A bolus is given to bring the plasma concentration back up to the target concentration and an infusion is then started to maintain the plasma and effect-site concentrations at the target concentration.

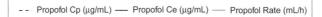

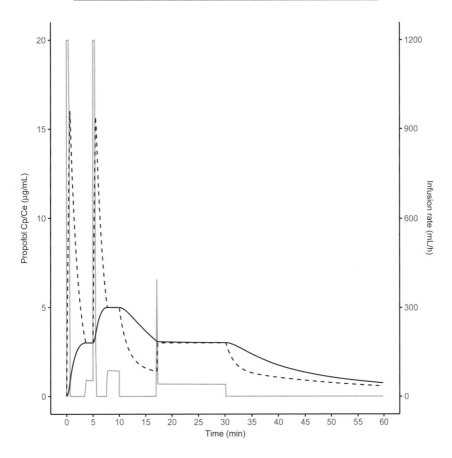

Figure 5: Effect-site targeted TCI using the Eleveld model. At time zero the target is set at 3 µg/ml, at 5 minutes it is increased to 5 µg/ml, and at 10 minutes it is reduced to 3 µg/ml. The target is set to zero at 40 minutes. At each target change the system manipulates the plasma concentration to rapidly achieve the target concentration.

Anaesthetists planning to use an effect-site targeted system need to bear in mind the fact that there are layers of assumptions inherent in effect-site targeting. Pharmacokinetic parameters and models, based on population studies, may not apply to an individual, and measured plasma concentrations may be quite different to those predicted. The choice of k_{eo} value used is especially critical in effect-site targeting, because it will determine the overshoot and undershoot in plasma concentrations used to steer the effect-site concentration when the target effect-site concentration is increased or decreased respectively. If two different systems use the same pharmacokinetic data set, but with different k_{eo} values, different drug doses will be administered leading to different peak and trough plasma concentrations. A "slower" k_{eo} value (i.e. a smaller rate constant) will cause a higher peak plasma concentration when the target concentration is increased and a deeper trough when the target is decreased.

In summary it is very important that a fixed k_{eo} should only be used for effect-site targeting when both kinetic and dynamic models have been calculated from the same study population. If this is not possible, then a TTPE algorithm should be used.

2

Pharmacokinetics

Pharmacokinetics is often described as the study of "what the body does to the drug". In essence pharmacokinetics describes the relationship between the dose administered in mass or molar units, and the resulting blood or plasma concentration. The microprocessor in TCI devices is programmed with an infusion algorithm that uses a pharmacokinetic model for the drug in use to calculate required infusion rates.

What is a pharmacokinetic model and how is it derived?

Pharmacokinetic models are mathematical models that can be used to predict the plasma concentration profile of a drug after a bolus dose or an infusion of varying duration. TCI systems apply "compartmental models" in the sense that the model comprises one or more virtual volumes. For a simple one-compartment model, the administered drug is considered to be uniformly distributed throughout that compartment, and then cleared (usually by metabolism) from it in an exponential fashion ("exponential" in the sense that a fixed proportion of the drug is removed by metabolism in each unit of time, so that the actual amount of drug removed depends on the concentration). When there are two or more compartments, then the model also incorporates methods of estimating the rates of transfer between the compartments.

They are typically derived by studying the relationship among administered dose, patient or subject measurable or observable characteristics ("co-variates" such as gender, age, weight or height), and measured plasma concentrations. The measured drug concentrations – either arterial or venous – are typically acquired from de novo studies in which the drug is administered to a group of patients or volunteers in a simple manner – a bolus or an infusion or both, is administered. Sometimes, more complex methods are used (e.g. TCI administration of the drug using an older model).[59]

Having acquired plasma concentrations measured after a known drug infusion regimen, investigators then typically apply non-linear mixed effects modelling techniques using software such as NONMEM ® (ICON, Dublin, Ireland) to develop a population model. Multiple iterative steps are involved in this process. Initially the most simple model structure is used, and a model generated for each subject in the study population. The investigator then attempts to develop a single population model that predicts the model parameters of an individual. Attempts are made to find covariates – observed characteristics of the participants in an experiment, such as gender, age, weight or height – that correlate with the model parameters. The model is made increasingly complex by adding co-variates, using different methods of adjusting the model parameter according to the co-variates, and eventually, adding additional compartments. Multiple ways can be tried to adjust model parameters according to age, weight or height. For any given co-variate (e.g. weight) a model parameter could be fixed (i.e. no correlation with weight) or it could be scaled using either a linear, log-linear, sigmoid, or power function. Allometric scaling, is a special case of a power function. It is applied to clearance, often with weight to the power 0.75.[60]

At each step, the model fit is evaluated, to determine the accuracy with which the model predicts the measured plasma concentrations of the subjects in the study (i.e. within-sample measurements), and statistical processes are applied to determine whether the new co-variate or new compartment improves model performance. If model performance is not significantly improved, then the investigator reverts to the more simple ('parsimonious') model. This continues until all avenues have been explored. Interested readers may wish to consult the detailed description we provided of the application of this technique to the development of the Eleveld general purpose propofol model.[57]

The kinetics of most of the currently used anaesthetic drugs can be described with reasonable accuracy by one or more two or three compartment models. Appendix 1 lists the model parameters for several commonly used anaesthetic agents. Each model describes the number of compartments, and their volumes, the rate of drug metabolism or elimination, and the rate of transfer of drug between the different compartments. The concept is summarised in Figure 2. By convention the compartment into which the drug is injected is called the central compartment (V1 or Vc). This is also referred to as the initial volume of distribution. The second compartment, V2 , is referred to as the "vessel-rich" or "fast distribution" compartment (because there is rapid drug distribution between V1 and V2), while the third compartment, V3, is referred to as the "vessel-poor" or "slow" compartment (because there is slow drug distribution between V1 and V3). The sum of V1, V2 and V3 gives the "volume of distribution at steady state," Vd_{ss}.

The central compartment may be thought of as including the blood or plasma volume, but note that the volume V1 may be larger than the blood or plasma volume. It is important to remember that the "volumes" of a two or three compartment model are theoretical volumes that can be used to predict plasma concentrations – they have no real anatomical or physiological correlates.

The rates of drug metabolism and distribution can be interchangeably described by rate constants or clearances. A rate constant describes a proportion of drug in a compartment undergoing a process during a unit of time, and is thus reported with the units min^{-1} or hr^{-1}. By convention we use the symbol k_{10} to denote the rate constant for metabolism or elimination, whereas the symbols k_{12}, k_{21}, k_{13} and k_{31} are used to denote the rate constants for drug transfer between V1 and V2, between V2 and V1, between V1 and V3, and between V3 and V1 respectively.

A brief example seeking to explain rate constants follows. If for drug X, the rate constants k_{13} and k_{31} are 0.05 and 0.005 respectively, this means that in each unit of time 5% of the total amount of drug X in compartment 1 moves into compartment 3, whereas 0.5% of the amount of drug X in compartment 3 moves into compartment 1 in each unit of time. Clearly the net movement of drug X, in mass or molar units, depends on the relative concentrations of drug X in the two compartments. If, for example, compartment 1 has a volume of 10 litres and the concentration of drug X at time zero is 1 µg/ml, then the amount of drug moving from compartment 1 to compartment 3 in the next minute is 500 µg (5% × 1 µg/ml × 10,000 ml). As can be seen below it follows from the ratio of the rate constants that the volume of compartment 3 must be 100 litres (10 litres × 0.05/0.005). If the concentration in this compartment happens to be 0.1 µg/ml at time zero, then the amount of drug moving from compartment 3 to compartment 1 is 50µg (0.5% of 10,000 µg) and so the net result is an overall movement of 450 µg of drug X from compartment 1 to compartment 3.

Clearances on the other hand describe a volume (of a compartment) that is "cleared" during a unit of time. The units are thus ml/min or ml/hr. If the compartment volume and the rate constants are known the clearances are easily calculated as follows:

Elimination clearance $= V1 \times k_{10}$

Clearance 2 $= V2 \times k_{21}$

Clearance 3 $= V3 \times k_{31}$

Sometimes when models are reported in the literature, only V_1 and the various rate constants are listed. This is because V_2 and V_3 can be deduced from the rate constants as follows:

$$V_2 = V_1 \times k_{12}/k_{21}$$
$$V_3 = V_1 \times k_{13}/k_{31}$$

Which model applies to my patient?

In modern clinical practice anaesthetists administer intravenous drugs for analgesia, sedation and anaesthesia to patients with a wide variety of characteristics that influence the pharmacokinetics and pharmacodynamics of the drugs being used. Factors of relevance include size, age and physiological status. Age is relevant because of the associated changes in size, and is particularly relevant in very young children (neonates) because the enzyme systems responsible for metabolising many drugs are underdeveloped at birth, and only 'mature' after the first few months of life. Size is important because it influences the volumes of distribution of our drugs, and with increasing obesity the relative sizes of the blood volume, muscle and adipose tissues changes disproportionately, all of which influence the rates of metabolism and distribution. Advancing age is also associated with relative changes in muscle and fat mass.

Many current models, and particularly those used for TCI, were developed from the data from studies in which a single drug was administered to volunteers or patients with a narrow range of characteristics (particularly age, weight, height and ASA status). For example, the Marsh and Schnider models for propofol, and the Minto model for remifentanil were developed from studies involving healthy adults, whereas the Paedfusor and Kataria propofol models were developed from data from children.[52-56 61-63] These models are thus only relevant to, and reasonably accurate in, patients with similar characteristics, receiving only that drug. The user of a TCI pump programmed with multiple models for a single drug thus has to choose the most appropriate model for the patient.

The 'Open TCI' project[1] provided an initial platform for researchers to share their data, and this helped to facilitate the development of so-called general purpose models developed from data from subjects with a broad variety of age, weight and height characteristics. It also enabled the incorporation of data from volunteers (who generally received a single drug) and from patients (who gener-

---

1 http://opentci.org/ (accessed 29 April 2019)

ally received other drugs which can significantly influence the pharmacokinetics of the drug being studied). This work has resulted in the development of general purpose models for propofol[57] and remifentanil[64] (see below). It is hoped that the availability in TCI pumps of these models, which are applicable in almost all patients, will simplify the operation of the pumps and enhance safety.

Pharmacokinetics of commonly used anaesthetic agents

We have recently reviewed the pharmacokinetics and dynamics of propofol in detail.[65]

POPULATION-SPECIFIC PROPOFOL MODELS

Adults

The three compartment model published by Marsh at al.[52] is used in the Diprifusor microprocessor ® (AstraZeneca, Macclesfield, UK) which is incorporated in all first generation TCI pumps, and is also available in second generation TCI pumps. It was pragmatically adapted from the model published by Gepts et al.[66] The publication in which the model parameters were first presented was actually a report of a study of the performance of the adult model in children, followed by the results of a prospective study of a new model specific for children (developed from retrospective analysis of the data from the earlier study).[52]

In the Marsh model the compartment volumes are linear functions of patient weight, and the rate constants are fixed. Accordingly the clearances are weight-related. Although the Marsh model parameters do not vary with age, as a safety feature the Diprifusor software requires the user to enter the patient age at start-up, and will not function if an age < 16 is entered.

In the early 2000's White et al. adapted the Marsh model to include age as a co-variate of V_1 and metabolic clearance (the effect is larger for females), but this version of the model has not been incorporated in commercially available TCI pumps.[67]

Studies in the late 1990s demonstrated that age, gender, height, mode of administration (bolus versus infusion) and site of blood sampling (venous versus arterial) all influence the pharmacokinetic model parameters. Schüttler et al. analysed the data from 9 studies of propofol pharmacokinetics in adults and children and produced a model that incorporates all the aforementioned factors and is valid for patients of all ages.[68] All model parameters except for V_3 calculated using a power function of body weight.

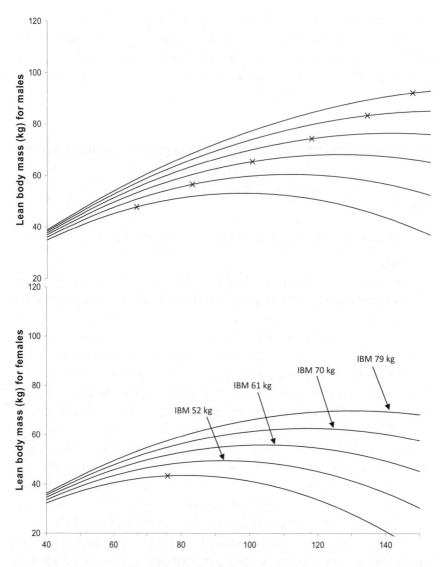

Figure 6: Relationship between body weight, height, lean and ideal body weight (LBM and IBW) for males (top panel) and females (lower panel). Each line shows the change in LBM for a given height (indicated on the right). IBWs for each height are indicated by crosses or text and arrows (when IBW does not fall on the LBM curve).

Schnider et al. followed a combined PK/PD approach to develop a model that is used for adult propofol administration in many second generation TCI pumps. It has a fixed V_1, age is a co-variate in the calculation of V_2 and Clearance 2, and height, total body weight, and lean body mass (LBM) are co-variates for the metabolic (elimination) clearance.[53][54] LBM is calculated with the James equation which is a quadratic function of height and weight (slightly different versions for males and females).[69] James developed these equations in the 1970s, when there was a lower incidence of severe obesity. For females of any given height, the LBM calculation reaches a maxima when the body mass index is ~37 kg/m^2. If the total body weight increases further, then the LBM paradoxically decreases. For males the maximum calculated LBM is reached with a BMI of ~42 kg/m^2.

Obese adults

Obesity is associated with complex changes in the pharmacokinetics of propofol, which were described in detail in a review published in 2007.[70] Servin showed that whereas the initial volume of distribution (V1) and distribution clearance are similar in obese and non-obese patients, the volume of distribution at steady state (sum of V1, V2 and V3) and the total body clearance of propofol do correlate with total body weight.[71] The Marsh and Schnider models both perform sub-optimally in obese subjects,[72] but for different reasons.[70] Over the years several models specifically designed for use in obese patients have been developed. Examples include the models developed by Dyck,[73] Wietasch,[72] van Kralingen [74] and Cortinez. [75]

Children

The pharmacokinetics of propofol differ significantly between children and adults.[76] [77] A study of the accuracy of target-controlled infusions using the Marsh adult model in 20 children found the model significantly overestimated plasma concentrations (i.e. measured plasma concentrations were lower than expected).[52] The Marsh model was then adapted to produce a model specific to children (the size of the central compartment volume was increased, but remained a linear function of body weight), and when prospectively tested, the predictive performance was better than when the adult model was used.[52]

Since then several other models specific to children have been produced.[78] Two of these models are commercially used for TCI administration in children. The three compartmental Kataria model was developed using three different pharmacokinetic modelling techniques in an extended group of children between 3 and 11 years.[61] It has fixed rate constants, while compartmental volumes have a linear correlation with weight. The Paedfusor model was adapted from one of the preliminary models developed by Schüttler prior to the publication of his final model.[68] The compartment volumes have a linear with weight, and distribution rate constants are fixed, whereas the metabolic rate constant, and therefore also clearance, is a power function of weight. In the final Schüttler model all variables have a non-linear correlation with age and weight. See Appendix for a detailed description of the models.

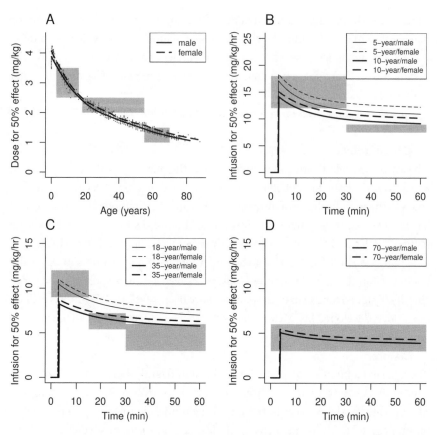

Figure 7: Predicted initial dose for 50% drug effect vs age for all of the individuals studied and maintenance infusion rates over time for illustrative children (5 yr, 18 kg, and 109 cm; 10 yr, 32 kg, 139 cm), adults (18 and 35 yr, 70 kg, and 170 cm), and elderly (70 yr, 70 kg, and 170 cm) individuals, assuming concomitant opioid administration. Induction and maintenance dosing recommendations for anaesthesia from the propofol package insert are shown in the shaded areas. Both the initial dose and maintenance infusion rates are generally close to recommended with smooth interpolation across the age range. (Modified from Eleveld et al. BJA 2018, 120, 942-959, with permission).

THE ELEVELD GENERAL PURPOSE PROPOFOL MODEL

Second generation TCI pumps were commonly programmed with one or more of the Marsh, Schnider, Paedfusor and Kataria models. This generates potential sources of error. Recent and future TCI pumps may also include a general purpose model for propofol (the so-called "Eleveld model"[57]). The reader should please note that the model incorporated in the pumps is the combined PK/PD model published in the British Journal of Anaesthesia in 2018 [57] which includes PD components, and a PK parameter data set is an updated and improved version of the preliminary Eleveld PK model published in Anesthesia and

Analgesia in 2014.[79] Eleveld developed the combined PK/PD model, using non-linear mixed effect modelling with data obtained from 30 previously published studies, five of which also contained BIS observations. Weight, age, post-menstrual age (PMA), height, sex, BMI, and presence/absence of concomitant opiates were explored as covariates. To cope with differences in size, distribution clearances are allometrically scaled with weight (using a power exponent of 0.75). Maturation effects in small children are dealt with by incorporating a sigmoid function in the calculation of V1, metabolic clearance and slow distribution clearance. The predictive performance of the model was evaluated in data from young children, children, adults, elderly, and high-BMI individuals, and in simulated TCI applications. Internal within sample testing showed similar or better performance than that of specialist models designed for specific sub-populations (children, elderly and obese).

The model has also been validated against the recommended dosing schemes from the propofol package insert and as shown in Figure 7. Predicted initial dose and maintenance infusion rates when targeting an effect-site concentration achieving accurate levels of anaesthesia or sedation are generally close to recommended with smooth interpolation across the age range.

The PD (pharmacodynamic) part of the model is connected to the PK model by a sigmoidal Emax PD model.[57] This allows a complete description of the dose-effect relationship and the correct use of effect-compartment controlled TCI techniques.

POPULATION-SPECIFIC REMIFENTANIL MODELS

Adults

Remifentanil is a synthetic opioid that is ultra- short-acting because it is metabolised by non-specific esterases present in most tissues of the body. This contrasts with most other anaesthetic agents first need to be present in the blood passing through the hepatic circulation before they can be inactivated by hepatic metabolism. Remifentanil pharmacokinetics are thus not modified by hepatic [80] or renal failure.[81]

TCI pumps currently incorporate the three compartment remifentanil model described by Minto for use in adults.[55][56] Co-variates include weight, height and gender (from which lean body mass are calculated), and age (see Appendix). Note the small sizes of the compartments and the relatively large rate constants for metabolism and re-distribution.

Obese adult models

To the best of our knowledge no remifentanil models have been specifically developed for use in obese patients.

Children

Rigby-Jones et al. and Ross et al. studied the pharmacokinetics of remifentanil in children. Rigby-Jones et al. studied a cohort of 26 neonates and children undergoing sedation with midazolam and remifentanil infusions after cardiac surgery. They found that a two compartment model, with metabolic and distribution clearances scaled allometrically with weight, best described the data.[82] Ross studied a cohort of 42 children ranging in age from 5 days to 17 years. The children each received a single 5 µg/kg bolus of remifentanil administered over 1 minute. They only reported non-compartmental parameters, but showed age-related effects on volume of distribution and clearance.[83]

GENERAL PURPOSE MODELS FOR REMIFENTANIL

La Colla et al. made a simple adaptation to the Minto model and studied the performance of the adapted model in an obese patient group.[84] The change made was to substitute the James equation (for calculating LBM) with the Janmahasatian equation [85] (which calculates lean body weight more accurately than the James equation, certainly in very short and obese patients). They found that this adapted model performed well in obese and in non-obese adult patients. This model has not been validated in children, to the best of our knowledge.

Kim et al.[86] developed a general purpose **adult** model from the combined data from 9 studies, of which two enrolled only obese patients [84][87] and one study obese and non-obese patients.[88] The model has a complex structure, with V1 scaling allometrically with total weight, V2 scales allometrically with fat-free mass whereas it decreases linearly with age, V3 does not scale with size but does decrease linearly with age, metabolic clearance scales allometrically with total weight and decreases linearly with age, fast distribution clearance decreases linearly with age, age slow distribution clearance is fixed. Within sample assessment of model performance showed that performance was similar to that of the La Colla and Minto models in the non-obese and elderly patients, whereas performance was much better than that of La Colla and Minto in the obese.

Eleveld developed a more generally applicable model across a wide age range.[64] He combined the data from two adult studies (Minto [55][56] and Mertens[89]) and the paediatric study of Ross,[83] but did not include data from obese patients. The kinetics of remifentanil were best described by a 3 compartmental model in which the volumes were scaled linearly with fat-free mass, but decrease with age, and clearances scaled allometrically with the estimated compartmental volumes.

SUFENTANIL

Sufentanil is a potent synthetic opioid whose pharmacokinetics are best described by a three compartment model, with a large volume of distribution (V3 is particularly large) but also a moderately fast metabolic clearance. Although suitable for use by infusion, it should be remembered that the kinetics are context-sensitive.[90] If it is infused for more than a couple of hours at clinically used target concentrations, the infusion should be stopped at least an hour before the end of the surgical procedure, to reduce the chances of a long delay before emergence and return to spontaneous breathing.

TCI pumps tend to incorporate the three compartment model developed by Gepts.[91] It has fixed compartmental volumes and fixed rate constants (i.e. compartment volumes and clearances are not affected by weight). Age does not appear to influence the pharmacokinetics of sufentanil. Although the model performs well in clinical practice, it should be noted that the data from which the model has been derived (and resulted in a cavoriate free model) was limited.

ALFENTANIL

Alfentanil is ± less fat-soluble than many other anaesthetic drugs. It is metabolised in the liver, but has a relatively low extraction ratio of 0.3 – 0.5.[92-94] Various compartmental models for alfentanil were developed in the early 1980's, but usually without using a formal population modelling approach.[92 93 95 96] Maitre however then applied NONMEM to the original data sets from these 4 above studies.[97] The resulting three compartmental model is the most commonly used model for TCI alfentanil systems. It incorporates weight, age and gender as co-variables in the calculation of compartment volumes and elimination and distribution rate constants. The model is characterised by small compartmental volumes, and a relatively small elimination rate constant (see Appendix for a list of the model parameters).

FENTANYL

The pharmacokinetics of fentanyl are best described by a three compartment model. Currently only a small number of commercially available pumps can be used for TCI administration of fentanyl, using the Shafer model.[33] His model was developed from a study of the predictive performance of previously developed fentanyl models.[98-100] The Shafer model has no covariates, but was developed from a cohort of non-obese patients. Shibutani and coworkers showed that the Shafer model systematically overpredicts plasma concentrations in obese patients, and suggested methods of improving predictive accuracy such as use of a "pharmacokinetic mass" or "dosing mass" calculated from total body weight, or an adjustment factor applied to the target concentration.[101]

Fentanyl is highly lipid soluble, and this results in a large VDss. Nonetheless, the clinical effects of commonly used single bolus doses (1.5 μg/kg) is only about 30 minutes (i.e. longer than that of alfentanil but shorter than that of morphine). As with alfentanil, the duration of effect is curtailed by rapid distribution. Despite the clinical impression that fentanyl produces a rapid onset, the time to peak effect is ~3.5 minutes, because of the rather slow equilibration time between plasma and the brain. Fentanyl undergoes extensive hepatic metabolism, producing inactive metabolites. Less than 10% of fentanyl is excreted unchanged in the urine. It is metabolized by hepatic P-450 enzymes (CYP3A) and so is susceptible to interactions with drugs that influence enzyme activity.

The lungs also serve as a large, inactive storage site, with an estimated 75% of the initial fentanyl dose undergoing first-pass pulmonary uptake.[102] This combined with its large volume of distribution (V3 is particularly large) is the reason why when infusions of fentanyl are administered, the context-sensitive half-time increases dramatically over time.[99] For similar reasons repeated boluses can cause a prolonged duration of effect.

DEXMEDETOMIDINE

We have recently reviewed the pharmacokinetics and pharmacodynamics of dexmedetomidine in detail.[103] In brief, the kinetics are somewhat slower than those of propofol. Dexmedetomidine is highly protein bound and although the compartment volumes are somewhat smaller than those in propofol models, metabolic clearance is relatively slow, meaning that dexmedetomidine accumulates more than propofol, causing an increase in context-sensitive half time as the duration of infusion increases. About 1% of dexmedetomidine is excreted unchanged, mostly in the urine. The remaining 99% of administered drug is eliminated by hepatic metabolism (by either glucuronidation by uridine diphosphate glucuronosyltransferase enzymes or by hydroxylation mediated by cytochrome P450 enzymes – mainly CYP2A6). The hepatic extraction ratio is 0.7 meaning that metabolism is dependent on liver blood flow.

Several adult pharmacokinetic models for dexmedetomidine have been developed, mostly from small studies involving postoperative ICU patients[104-111] or healthy volunteers.[59 112 113] The Dyck model was developed from a study involving 10 volunteers.[114] Metabolic clearance scales linearly with height, but all other parameters are fixed. Hannivoort and Colin used this model to administer dexmedetomidine by TCI twice (two sessions separated by at least a week) to 16 volunteers.[59] Measured dexmedetomidine concentrations were then used to generate a new, optimized model. A three compartment model with volumes linearly scaled to total weight, and clearance allometrically scaled to total weight (exponent 0.75). As the investigators also simultaneously recorded various clinical effects and haemodynamic effects in this study, a combined PK-PD model could be developed. Using the "Hannivoort-Colin model", the user will be able to obtain information on the effect-site concentration of dexmedetomidine.[115 116]

Cortinez et al. studied the effects of obesity on dexmedetomidine pharmacokinetics in two patient studies.[106 117] In the first study they found that the data were best explained by a two compartment model in which the volumes scaled linearly with fat-free mass, whereas the clearance scaled allometrically with FFM.[106] They also found that metabolic clearance declined with increasing fat mass. In a subsequent study,[117] also in obese and non-obese patients, dexmedetomidine was administered based on lean body weight measured by dual X-ray absorptiometry, and then assessed the effect on metabolic clearance of different weight parameters, liver blood flow (measured by ICG clearance), and UGT gene expression. They again found that the data were best described by a two compartment model with volumes scaled linearly with lean body weight, but this time found that metabolic clearance co-varied best with liver blood flow, and was not affected by the other factors studied.

TCI administration has been used in several studies.[59 108 114 118] It is important to remember that the dexmedetomidine loading dose should always be given slowly (i.e. over 10 minutes) to avoid serious cardiovascular adverse effects. As TCI pumps will soon incorporate a model for dexmedetomidine it will therefore be necessary for the pump manufacturers to implement an algorithm to limit the maximum infusion rate limitation during administration of the (initial) dexmedetomidine bolus.[59 115 116]

Paediatric dexmedetomidine models

Several groups have studied the pharmacokinetics of dexmedetomidine in children, although this has mostly been done in critically ill children,[119 120] or children and neonates undergoing sedation after cardiac surgery.[121 122] Another group has studied a more general surgical population of children.[123] All have found that a two compartment model with allometric scaling of clearances best describes the data, and several have shown evidence of maturation effects in metabolic clearance.[120 124 125]

KETAMINE

Ketamine is available as either a racemic mixture of the R(-) and S(+) isomers, or a formulation containing only the S(+) isomer (commonly known as esketamine). Although pharmacokinetics of the two isomers are somewhat different,[126-133] both isomers are highly lipid soluble, with large volumes of distribution, but with fast distribution clearance, which is why single bolus dose are associated with a short duration of action, and also rapid metabolic clearance. The racemic mixture and esketamine are both well-suited to use by infusion. Both isomers are metabolized by the liver, mostly by demethylation to norketamine (which is ~20% as active as ketamine), followed by hydroxylation to hydroxynorketamine. Finally glucuronidation occurs rendering a water-soluble that is excreted in the urine.

TCI technology has been used for ketamine administration in studies in different settings, including critical care,[134 135] the operating theatre,[133 136] and neuroscience studies.[137-140] The three compartment Domino model [128] (see Appendix) is the most commonly used model for TCI ketamine administration. Several other three compartment models for the ketamine enantiomers,[130 131 133] and two compartment models for ketamine [135 141] have been published.

Accuracy of target-controlled infusion systems

A TCI system administers a drug at changing infusion rates that are determined by a mathematical algorithm that uses a model derived from studies of the pharmacokinetics of that drug in a population of patients or subjects. It is important to remember that the concentration shown on the user interface is only an estimate. Many factors can influence the actual drug concentrations achieved. Thanks to technological developments and strict regulatory controls, technical factors (such as the accuracy of the motors that drive infusion pumps and correct microprocessor programming to ensure proper implementation of pharmacokinetic models) are unlikely to be significant.[142] More relevant factors are whether or not the drug is actually reaching the intravascular space (there may be a line disconnection or the intravenous cannula may not be in a vein) and whether or not the pharmacokinetic model in use applies to the individual patient.

Before a model can be used clinically it should undergo clinical validation to assess the predictive accuracy of the model in one or more groups of subjects. Ideally this should be a prospective study in which the model is used to control an infusion of the drug, and plasma concentrations are then measured and compared with the predicted concentrations. Model performance is sometimes assessed "retrospectively" by using data from a study in which another model is used to control the infusion, the infusion rates and volumes are recorded, and drug concentrations measured. This enables the researchers to then "back calculate" the concentrations estimated by other models and compare these estimations with the measured concentrations.

Finally, another method of validation of a model is to use it to calculate the bolus size and infusion rates required to reach and maintain an appropriate effect-site concentration, and to then compare the bolus size and subsequent infusion rates with those recommended in the SPC (summary of product characteristics, which is provided as the 'package insert' for every drug). This approach, was also applied to the Eleveld PK/PD model, as mentioned above (also see figure 7).[57]

In 1992 Varvel and colleagues proposed a set of standard criteria for assessing the predictive performance of computerised infusion pumps.[143] These criteria are MDPE (median performance error, a measure of bias or offset), MDAPE (median absolute performance error, a measure of inaccuracy or imprecision), wobble (a measure of the intra-individual variability in errors) and divergence (a measure of any trend over time in the size and magnitude of errors). To calculate these criteria it is necessary to first calculate the performance error (PE) for each measured drug concentration, C_{meas}, where the calculated or predicted concentration is C_{pred}, as follows:

For the jth measurement in the ith patient:

$$PE_{ij} = \frac{(C_{meas} - C_{pred})}{C_{pred}} \times 100$$

The four criteria are then calculated as follows:
For the ith patient for whom N_i drug assays were performed
$$MDPE_i = \text{Median} [PE_{ij}, j = 1, ..., N_i]$$
$$MDAPE_i = \text{Median} [|PE_{ij}|, j = 1, ..., N_i]$$
$$Wobble_i = \text{Median} [|PE_{ij} - MDPE_i|, j = 1, ..., N_i]$$

Divergence: is calculated for each individual as the slope of the linear regression of that individual's absolute performance errors over time (a positive value indicates that the performance errors are increasing over time, whereas a negative value indicates that the measured values are converging with the predicted values over time)

For computer-controlled infusion pumps a MDPE (bias) of 10 – 20 % and a MDAPE of 20 – 40 % have been proposed as acceptable.[144 145] These figures can be put into perspective by considering end-tidal volatile agent monitoring. Standard teaching holds that the end-tidal concentration of a volatile anaesthetic agent is equivalent to the arterial tension of the anaesthetic agent. Studies comparing the end-tidal and measured arterial concentrations of isoflurane have shown that the difference between the two depends on the phase of the anaesthetic – being greatest during induction and emergence – but is commonly of the order of 20% during the maintenance phase.[146 147]

So how well do the different pharmacokinetic models match up to these standards? A full discussion of the performance of all the models for the drugs mentioned above is beyond the scope of this booklet. Naturally the best performing models tend to be the ones most commonly used. In the following section the performance of the "better" models will be highlighted.

PROPOFOL

Adult

The two main models currently in use are those described by Marsh[52] and Schnider[53 54].

A small number of studies have prospectively evaluated the predictive performance of the Marsh model when it is used for propofol TCI. Swinhoe showed that the predictive performance of the model was similar in young (18 – 40 years), middle-aged (41 – 55 years) and elderly (56 – 80 years) patients, with an overall bias (MDPE) of 16% and overall inaccuracy (MDAPE) of 24%.[44] In 10 young healthy adult patients Coetzee et al. found a MDPE of –7% and a MDAPE of 18%.[73] In adults undergoing coronary artery surgery, Barvais found MDPE of 21 and 10% during the pre-bypass on bypass periods respectively, and MDAPE values of 23 and 18% before and during bypass respectively.[43] In a study of underweight patients TCI propofol using the Marsh model, Lee et al. showed that the Marsh model over-predicted plasma concentrations – MDPE was -16% and MDAPE 27%.[148]

As a secondary study outcome, Rigouzzo evaluated the predictive performance of the Schnider model in 45 subjects aged 14 to 32 years. They found that almost all measured propofol concentrations were higher than the predicted ones, but they did not report formal Varvel criteria.[149] In a study of propofol pharmacodynamics, Doufas studied the predictive performance of Schnider-based propofol TCI administration as a secondary goal, and showed MDPE of 1.8% and MDAPE of 21%.[150] We are only aware of one published study that was specifically designed to evaluate the predictive performance of the Schnider model during TCI propofol administration using the Schnider model. This was the above-mentioned study of Lee and colleagues, in which a cohort of underweight patients received Schnider-based TCI propofol administration.[148] They showed that in these patients the Schnider model underestimated propofol concentrations, with a MDPE of 3% and MDAPE of 28%. Many more studies have evaluated and compared the predictive performance of these models in other situations, such as evaluation of the predictive performance of one model when propofol was administered at fixed infusion rates, or by TCI using another model. Sahinovic and co-workers compared the PK and PD of propofol in patients about to undergo brain tumour excision, with patients about to undergo spinal surgery.[151] Patients initially received fixed infusion rates, and later Schnider TCI. In the spinal surgery group the MDPE and MDAPE were 8.6 and 41% for the Marsh model and 1.9 and 18% for the Schnider model. For the tumour group MDPE and MDAPE were -14 and 41% for the Marsh model and -20 and 23% for the Schnider model.

Recently, during the development of the Eleveld model, we analysed the predictive performance of the Marsh and Schnider models in a large pooled data set comprising propofol pharmacokinetic data from all published studies for which the raw data were available.[79] Subjects in these data sets received propofol administration via a variety of methods (fixed infusion rates, TCI administration using different models). In this data set the MDPE and MDAPE of the Schnider model among non-obese and non-elderly adults was 2.1 and 26%, and that of the Marsh model 12 and 23%. The performance of the preliminary Eleveld model in the same group was -0.8 and 21.5%. The Eleveld model performed significantly better than the Marsh and Schnider models (and better than the specialist models) at predicting propofol concentrations in the elderly and obese patients.

Children

Studies of the predictive performance of the Marsh model in children have shown that it over-predicts plasma concentrations (bias is of the order of −20%, meaning that measured concentrations tend to be 20% lower than those calculated by the system).[52][152] The revised Marsh (paediatric) model showed a far better bias,[62] as did the Short model which showed bias of −0.1% and precision of 21.5%.[152] The Paedfusor model performed very well when it was studied in 29 children undergoing cardiac surgery or cardiac catheterisation – bias was 4.1% and precision 9.7%.[62] There are no peer-reviewed publications of prospective studies of the predictive performance of the Kataria model.

In the above-mentioned 'Eleveld' data set, the Eleveld model performed significantly better than the Kataria and Paedfusor models. In children (age 3 – 18 years) the Eleveld model MDPE and MDAPE were -3.7 and 19.3% and in small children (age <3 years) the same performance parameters were -3.8 and 18.0%.[79]

More recently Hara et al. studied the performance of 11 different models during long duration manually controlled infusions of propofol in children.[78] In their population all models were associated with a negative bias. The best performing model was that developed by Short [152] (MDPE -10.5 and MDAPE 17.5%).

REMIFENTANIL

Mertens and colleagues studied the predictive performance of several remifentanil models during propofol/remifentanil anaesthesia.[51] For the Minto model they found a bias of –15% and precision of 20%. Drover et al. studied the predictive performance of the Minto model in 40 patients undergoing abdominal surgery and found a similar precision (18.2%), but a much better bias of 1.59%.

In a retrospective study of predictive performance in 3 combined remifentanil data sets, MDPE and MDAPE among middle-aged adults was -3.0 and 20% for the Minto model, and 2.0 and 20% for the Eleveld remifentanil model.[64]

SUFENTANIL

Studies of the predictive performance of the Gepts model show acceptable bias and precision. Published MDPE values range between -2.3 and -22.3% and MDAPE values range between 20.7 and 29.0%. [153-155] In a study involving obese patients, the Gepts model performance indices were similar (MDPE –12.8% and MDAPE 19.8%).[156]

ALFENTANIL

Maitre et al. tested the predictive performance of his model in adult patients undergoing abdominal and superficial surgery, and found acceptable results: MDPE was -7.9 and MDAPE 22.3%.[157] However, when Barvais et al. studied several alfentanil models in elderly patients he found that the Maitre model tended to underpredict the plasma alfentanil concentration (i.e. bias or MDPE were positive) and the inaccuracy (MDAPE) was > 40%.[158]

FENTANYL

As mentioned previously Shafer found that the MDAPE for the McClain model was 61% whereas the MDAPE for the Scott model was 33%.[33] Shibutani and colleagues studied the predictive performance of the Shafer model in lean and obese patients,[101] and found that while the model performed reasonably well in lean patients, in the obese it systematically overpredicted plasma concentrations as total body mass increased. The authors examined various solutions to this problem, and recommended that clinicians who wish to use TCI fentanyl use the Shafer model as it is (none of the parameters are weight-adjusted), but make a fairly simple upward adjustment to the target concentration in the obese.[101]

KETAMINE

In a retrospective study of the predictive performance of the Domino model during 4 studies involving low-dose target-controlled ketamine infusions, performance was sub-optimal.[159] The model significantly overpredicted ketamine plasma concentrations for the first hour of infusion, and then after a further hour or so, and particularly after the infusion were stopped, it tended to underpredict ketamine concentrations.

Pharmacokinetic interactions

Pharmacokinetic interactions occur when the presence of one drug causes an alteration in the pharmacokinetics of another agent. They are common among anaesthetic agents, of which the interactions between propofol and various opioid agents are described in most detail. Proposed mechanisms for these interactions include competition between propofol and opioids for pulmonary binding sites,[160] inhibition by propofol of cytochrome P450,[161] and haemodynamic alterations caused by propofol.[162] It is also likely that at higher concentrations propofol alters its own metabolism by causing changes to cardiac output and hepatic blood flow.

When combinations of drugs are used the blood or plasma concentrations are slightly higher than expected – of the order of 15 – 40% greater (see below). While these interactions should be borne in mind, it is seldom necessary to alter the target concentrations used because of pharmacokinetic interactions. In contrast, the synergism arising from pharmacodynamic interactions among anaesthetic agents is of greater significance and commonly requires a decrease of target concentration.

PROPOFOL/FENTANYL

Cockshott et al. found that if 100 μg of fentanyl is given before a bolus of propofol, the subsequent propofol concentrations are 50% greater than expected.[163]

PROPOFOL/ALFENTANIL

Pavlin et al., when comparing propofol concentrations in subjects receiving propofol alone with those in subjects receiving both propofol and alfentanil infusions, found that a target alfentanil concentration of 40 ng/ml was associated with a 19 – 29% increase in propofol concentration.[164] In the same study, *alfentanil* concentrations were also significantly higher when it was infused with propofol than when it was infused alone.

Mertens and colleagues studied the pharmacokinetics of propofol in male volunteers and found significant reductions in elimination clearance (metabolism) and in inter-compartmental clearance rates for alfentanil in the presence of propofol.[162]

PROPOFOL/REMIFENTANIL

Bouillon and colleagues have shown that co-administration of propofol with remifentanil causes 41% decreases in the central compartment volume and distributional clearance, and a 15% decrease in the elimination clearance of remifentanil.[165] Remifentanil did not appear to alter the pharmacokinetics of propofol.

3
—
Pharmacodynamics

General

Pharmacodynamics describes the relationship between blood or plasma concentration of a drug and clinical effect; and so is often said to describe "what the drug does to the body."

A full description of the clinical pharmacodynamics of the anaesthetics is beyond the scope of this book. For more details on the mechanisms of action and clinical pharmacology of the drugs, it is best to consult recent versions of one or more textbooks.[166-168]

In the following section the scientific literature concerning the range of therapeutic concentrations for various drugs will be outlined. In a subsequent section (Practical aspects – induction and maintenance of anaesthesia) we will offer practical advice on TIVA practice and specifically on the choice of target concentrations. While reading the following section readers should note that no single regimen, concentration or drug combination applies to all patients, and that doses of drugs used should be titrated according to the clinical response of the patient.

Pharmacodynamics of commonly used anaesthetic agents

PROPOFOL

Propofol is a $GABA_A$ agonist, which is commonly used for sedation and anaesthesia. The clinical pharmacology of the drug has been summarised recently.[65]

Sedation

Propofol at low doses is associated with a pleasant feeling (bordering on euphoria), anxiolysis and sedation. The plasma and effect-site concentrations required to achieve these effects vary markedly among patients.

Propofol has potent amnesic effects, with amnesia even occurring at sub-sedative concentrations. Using a Trivial Pursuit learning task Leslie and colleagues found that a **measured** plasma propofol concentration of 0.66µg/ml inhibited learning in 50% of volunteers.[169]

Studies using patient-maintained sedation (PMS) systems provide objective evidence of the likely dose requirements for sedation, because they allow the patient to control the dose (target concentration of a TCI system). When patients used a PMS system to self-administer propofol for anxiolysis before and during surgery, median target plasma propofol concentration were 1.0 and 1.3 µg/ml and 0.8 – 0.9 µg/ml respectively (Marsh model estimations). [170 171]

More recently physician controlled TCI propofol (Marsh model) was used for sedation in 122 adult patients on 6 intensive care units (along with morphine, fentanyl or alfentanil for analgesia).[172] The median target propofol concentration used was 1.34 µg/ml in post-cardiac surgery patients, 0.98 µg/ml in brain injured adults and 0.42 µg/ml in general intensive care patients. The mean average propofol infusion rate was 1.8 mg/kg/hr (range 0.2 – 4.8 mg/kg/hr).

In a study of healthy volunteers who received gradually increasing doses of propofol, the estimated effect-site concentration (Schnider model) associated with a 50% probability of responsiveness to verbal command (EC50) was 2.9 µg/ml (95% CI 2.7–3.1) when only propofol was administered.[173] In another study of volunteers who received different combinations of propofol and remifentanil, among those only receiving propofol the EC50 for loss of responsiveness was 2.2 µg/ml and the EC50 for loss of responsiveness to oesophagoscopy 4.1 µg/ml, in both cases as estimated by the Schnider model.[174] Figure 8 (lower panel) shows the strong influence of age on the effect-site concentration estimated by the Schnider model, at which 50% of patients can be expected to lose verbal responsiveness.

As mentioned earlier, the PD element of the Eleveld propofol PK/PD model can be used to estimate the effect-site propofol concentrations required for different decreases in the BIS. Figure 8 (upper panel) shows the influence of age on the effect-site concentration expected to cause a decline in the BIS to 84, a level associated with conscious sedation. For a 40 year old individual, the Eleveld model estimated effect-site propofol concentration associated with a BIS of 84 is just under 1 µg/ml.

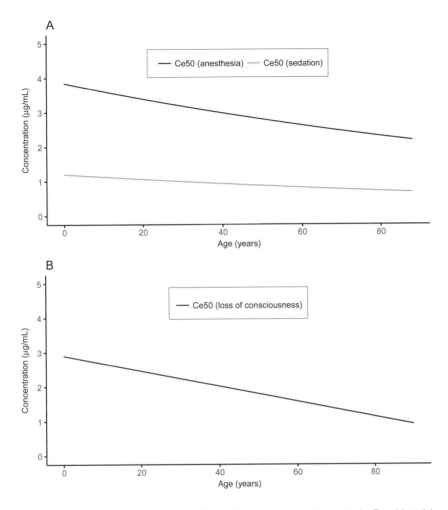

Figure 8: Upper panel: Age-dependent predicted effect-site concentrations with the Eleveld model to achieve 10 % and 50 % drug effect, being the accurate concentration for sedation (resulting in a population mean BIS of 84) and anaesthesia (resulting in a population mean BIS of 47). Lower panel: Age-dependent predicted effect-site concentrations using the Schnider model to "fall asleep".

Induction and maintenance of anaesthesia

Published data on measured plasma concentrations at loss and return of consciousness exist but are not very informative. The effect-site concentration of a drug cannot be directly measured, but is the concentration that largely determines the clinical effect, and large differences between the plasma and effect-site concentrations occur during the non-steady state conditions at induction of, and emergence from anaesthesia. Davidson for example reported EC50 values for measured propofol concentrations at loss of consciousness (8.1 µg/ml in patients only receiving propofol, and 5.4 µg/ml in patients receiving propofol and N_2O), but not estimated effect-site concentrations.[175]

In patients about to undergo spinal surgery Sahinovic found median (IQR) measured plasma propofol concentrations of 12.6 (11.5–15.1) µg/ml at loss of responsiveness.[176] These concentrations were rather similar to the predicted (Schnider model) estimations of plasma concentrations – 14.6 (13.4–15.2) µg/ml – but of course very different to the estimated effect-site concentrations at that time – 6.4 (5.2–7.8) µg/ml. During emergence the gradient between plasma and effect-site concentrations is usually smaller than that during induction. Measured plasma concentrations in the range 1.0 to 2.19 µg/ml have been recorded in volunteers on emergence from anaesthesia.[177] In the study of Sahinovic mentioned above, mean (IQR) measured plasma propofol concentrations at return of consciousness were 0.8 (0.6–1.1) µg/ml, estimated (Schnider model) plasma propofol concentrations were 0.9 (0.7–1.2) µg/ml, and estimated (Schnider model) effect-site propofol concentrations were 1.1 (0.8–1.4) µg/ml.

The following sections briefly summarise some of the data on target concentrations required for loss or and maintenance of anaesthesia with the different propofol models.

Marsh model

In unpremedicated patients in whom no other anaesthetic agents are administered, reported mean plasma propofol concentration required for induction of anaesthesia (loss of consciousness) are of the order of 5 – 6 µg/ml.[42 46] In patients who have received a sedative premedication or those in whom propofol is supplemented by nitrous oxide or an opioid, plasma concentrations in the range 4 – 5 µg/ml are required.[34 42 46]

During maintenance of anaesthesia the goals are to maintain unconsciousness, and to prevent responses to noxious stimuli. Propofol concentrations required to prevent a response to a noxious stimulus therefore give some indication of the concentrations required for maintenance of anaesthesia during surgical procedures. Studies by Stuart and Davidson found that the Marsh model estimated plasma propofol concentration required to prevent purposeful movement in response to surgical incision in 50% of patients (C_{p50}) is of the order of 6 – 7 µg/ml in un-premedicated patients not receiving nitrous oxide, and 4 – 5 µg/ml in un-premedicated patients receiving 67% nitrous oxide.[175 178] When opioids have also been administered, then the required propofol target concentrations will be significantly reduced (of the order of 50% – see the data below for the Schnider model).

Schnider model

Figure 8 shows the age-dependent EC50 concentration for "falling asleep" when using the Schnider model. Struys et al, using the Schnider model, found that the $Ce_{50, LOC}$ (effect-site propofol concentration required for loss of eyelash reflex in 50% of patients) was 2.9 μg/ml if only propofol was used, 1.8 μg/ml in the presence of remifentanil 2 ng/ml and 1.7 μg/ml in the presence of remifentanil 4 ng/ml.[173] In a study performed some years later, mentioned above, Sahinovic et al. studied propofol concentrations at loss and return of consciousness in patients with and without brain tumours.[176] Patients were given verbal command every 10 seconds. The moment of loss of consciousness was defined as the time when the patient failed to respond to a command for the second time. Median (IQR) estimated propofol effect-site concentrations in the non-tumour patients were 6.4 (5.2 – 7.8) μg/ml at the moment of loss of consciousness and 1.1 (0.8 – 1.4) μg/ml at return of consciousness. The estimated effect-site concentrations were similar in patients with tumours.

Struys and colleagues reported that the C_{e50} for preventing a response to noxious stimuli was 4.1 μg/ml when only propofol was used, 1.8 μg/ml when remifentanil 2 ng/ml was administered and 1.7 μg/ml when remifentanil 4 ng/ml was administered.[173]

Eleveld model

At present there are no published epidemiological data from prospective studies to show the range of Eleveld model estimated plasma and effect-site concentrations at loss and return of consciousness.

The model was, however, developed from a very large data set. Overall it comprised 15,433 measured propofol concentrations and 28,639 BIS observations from 1033 individuals (672 males and 361 females) with an age range from 27 weeks PMA to 88 years and a weight range from 0.68 to 160 kg. We are therefore confident that the model predictions of target concentrations required for loss and maintenance of consciousness – as shown in Figure 8 – are accurate and will be further validated in prospective studies.

As can be seen in Figure 8, the model estimates that for 20 year old individuals, an average effect-site concentration of 3.4 μg/ml is required for a BIS of 47, whereas for 40 year old individuals on average an effect-site concentration of 3.0 μg/ml is required, and for 80 year old individuals on average an effect-site concentration of 2.3 μg/ml is required. Our preliminary observations are that these target concentrations will usually be sufficient for induction and for maintenance of anaesthesia (i.e. target concentrations may not need to be significantly reduced after loss of consciousness as observed with some other models).[179] The propofol dose rates required to achieve these target effect-site concentrations fit very well within the dose recommendations of the figures mentioned in the SPC (summary of product characteristics) sheets supplied by the propofol manufacturers and approved by the regulatory authorities. This applies to the recommended bolus doses for induction and to infusion rates recommended for maintenance of anaesthesia, the children, non-obese adults, obese adults, and elderly patients (see Figure 7).

REMIFENTANIL

Remifentanil is a pure μ opioid receptor antagonist. Most of the published information refers to the use of remifentanil in association with TCI propofol or an inhalational agent for induction and maintenance of anaesthesia in ventilated adult patients. The remifentanil target concentrations used reflect the syngergistic pharmacodynamic interaction between remifentanil and hypnotic agents.[89] For most patients, a target concentration between 4 – 6 ng/ml will provide profound analgesia, prevent endotracheal tube induced coughing, and prevent movement responses to painful stimuli. Simulations using the Minto model show that in a 70 kg, 170 cm, 40 year old patient a remifentanil infusion rate of 0.25 μg/kg/min, will result in a plasma remifentanil concentration of about 6 ng/ml within 10 – 15 min.

Target concentrations >10 ng/ml are rarely needed, even during particularly stimulating surgery.

SUFENTANIL

Sufentanil has been used as a mono-anaesthetic agent during cardiac surgery, but for this very high plasma concentrations of sufentanil (> 20 ng/ml) are required.[180] In studies using TCI sufentanil with the Gepts model in combination of propofol, isoflurane or midazolam, the target plasma concentrations used were between 1 and 10 ng/ml during cardiac surgery [153][155] and between 0.1 and 1 ng/ml during general surgery.[154][156] The plasma concentration associated with a 50% probability of adequate spontaneous ventilation is 0.15 – 0.2 ng/ml and the concentration associated with a 50% probability of a response to skin incision or other painful stimuli is 0.3 – 0.4 ng/ml.[167]

In some countries, recommended concentrations are included in the drug label. In France the drug label recommends target concentrations between 0.4 and 2 ng/ml for cardiac surgery, and between 0.15 and 0.6 ng/ml for non-cardiac surgery.

ALFENTANIL

Alfentanil is approximately 10 times more potent than morphine. Numerous publications have described ranges of "therapeutic concentrations" for alfentanil. When used with nitrous oxide and no other hypnotic, Cp50 values of alfentanil for intubation and skin incision are 475 and 279 ng/ml respectively.[31 181 182] These high values reflect the low hypnotic potency of nitrous oxide.

Vuyk studied the pharmacodynamics of alfentanil as a supplement to either propofol or N_2O during lower abdominal surgery in female patients.[183] Fixed concentrations of either propofol (3 µg/ml) or nitrous oxide (66%) were administered, and the target concentration of alfentanil was adjusted according to patient responses. The Cp 50 values for alfentanil in combination with propofol were 92 ng/ml for intubation, 55 ng/ml for skin incision, 84 ng/ml for peritoneal incision, and 66 ng/ml for the intra-abdominal part of surgery. The corresponding values during nitrous oxide anaesthesia were significantly higher: 429 ng/ml for intubation, 101 ng/ml for skin incision, and 206 ng/ml for the intra-abdominal part of surgery.

FENTANYL

Fentanyl is approximately 100 fold more potent than morphine. As TCI fentanyl is not used clinically, the literature describing therapeutic concentrations mostly comes from older studies. Generally therapeutic plasma concentrations for fentanyl are reported to be between 1 and 3 ng/ml.[184-186]

KETAMINE

In volunteers receiving only ketamine, plasma concentrations of the order of 100 – 200 ng/ml were associated with adverse psychiatric effects.[137-140] The infusion rates for these plasma concentrations are of the order of 0.25 – 0.5 mg/kg/hr. When used as an analgesic adjunct during general anaesthesia for painful surgery, infusion rates of 0.25 mg/kg/hr are commonly used.

Ketamine is seldom used as the sole hypnotic agent because of the adverse emergence phenomena. Exceptions include circumstances such as battlefield anaesthesia, repeated procedures for burns, and anaesthesia in limited resource countries. Recently there has been a resurgence of interest in this drug as an anaesthetic and analgesic adjuvant. Potential benefits include neuroprotection,[187] pre-emptive analgesia, and attenuation of postoperative hyperalgesia.[188] However, a Cochrane review found only weak evidence of improved acute pain scores,[189] and a large recent multi-center study failed to show a reduction in postoperative pain scores and the incidence of delirium.[190]

DEXMEDETOMIDINE

For sedation, plasma and effect-site concentrations of between 0.6 and 1.2 ng/ml are required.[115] These concentrations are associated with infusion rates of roughly 0.5 – 1.0 µg/kg/hr.

Pharmacodynamic interactions

A pharmacodynamic interaction is said to occur when the use of a combination of agents results in a change in the clinical effect from that which would have occurred if either agent had been used on its own. Additive or supra-additive pharmacodynamic interactions between most classes of anaesthetic agents have been found. Opioids, benzodiazepines, clonidine and even esmolol have all been shown to reduce the dose requirements of intravenous and inhalational hypnotic agents.[184 191-201] In general, additive drug interactions occur when combining drugs acting by a similar mechanism and supra- or infra-additive interaction when combining drugs acting by a different mechanism.[202-204] **Pharmacodynamic** interactions tend to be far more significant, and potent, than **pharmacokinetic** interactions. The most widely studied anaesthestic interactions are those between opioids and various hypnotics.[205]

In the previous section we discussed the study by Vuyk et al. of the influence of propofol on the alfentanil dose required to prevent responses to intraoperative noxious stimuli. The same authors later performed another study of the pharmacodynamic interaction between propofol and alfentanil, during which the patients received one of four fixed concentrations of alfentanil, while propofol concentrations were adjusted.[206] It enabled them to determine plasma propofol concentrations associated with different end points, at different alfentanil concentrations. These endpoints included loss and return of consciousness, and 10% reductions in blood pressure and heart rates. A similar study has investigated the pharmacodynamic interaction between propofol and remifentanil (again examining responses to noxious stimuli, and concentrations associated with loss and return of consciousness).[89]

Using TCI with the Schnider and Minto model for propofol and remifentanil, respectively, Struys and colleagues found a similar degree of synergism for propofol and remifentanil with regard to loss of response to noxious stimuli during induction of anaesthesia.[173] They also examined the interaction with regard to loss of eyelash reflex, and loss of response to verbal command. As expected, given the potent analgesic effects of remifentanil, the synergism between remifentanil and propofol was most profound for response to painful stimuli – a remifentanil effect-site concentration of 4 ng/ml reduced the Ce50 for loss of response to verbal command from 2.9 to 2.2 µg/ml; whereas it reduced the Ce50 for loss of response to noxious stimulus from 4.1 to 1.3 µg/ml. What was more interesting and unexpected is that in the presence of a modest dose of remifentanil, the propofol Ce50 for response to pain was lower than that required for both response to verbal command and for loss of eyelash reflex.

Commonly, interactions between two drugs have been illustrated by drawing isobolograms – figures showing a line joining all pairs of concentrations of two drugs that result in the same effect (e.g. a 50% probability of response to a painful stimulus). Response surface models are the logical next step and have greatly improve our understanding of pharmacodynamics interactions among 2 [207] [208] or even 3 drugs.[209] The nature of the interaction may be different at different drug effect levels (for example additive at the 50% level but synergistic at the 95% level). Response surface models aim to characterize the response surface describing all levels of effect. They thus combine information about the full range of isoboles resulting from the concentration response curves of all combinations of the drugs involved.

Combinations of agents that result in supra-additive clinical effects offer significant benefits for patients. They enable the anaesthetist to achieve clinically equivalent levels of anaesthesia with lower total doses of drugs. In general the hypnotic agents (inhalational and intravenous) tend to have more profound effects on cardiovascular parameters (such as blood pressure, systemic resistance and cardiac output) than the opioids. Thus when a combination of a hypnotic and an opioid is used, the dose of hypnotic can be reduced to enhance cardiovascular stability, which is especially beneficial in patients with limited cardiac reserves.

Bouillon et al. subsequently studied the pharmacodynamic interaction between propofol and remifentanil, with the endpoints being response to shaking, shouting and laryngoscopy.[208] Their findings confirm the dramatic synergism between the two agents. While remifentanil alone did not ablate the responses to laryngoscopy, and even to shaking and shouting, propofol in higher doses was able to do so. Modest concentrations of remifentanil cause a large reduction in the target propofol concentrations required to ablate the responses. Using findings from Bouillon et al., van den Berg et al. explored whether four effect-site propofol and remifentanil combinations chosen from along the isobole that yields tolerance to laryngoscopy in 90 % of the patients, would result in favorable endpoints for immobility, haemodynamic stability and an adequate hypnotic drug effect as measured by EEG.[210] The pairs of effect-site target concentrations of propofol (Schnider) and remifentanil (Minto) were: 8.6 and 1, 5.9 and 2, 3.6

and 4 and 2.0 and 8 ug/ml and ng/ml, respectively. They concluded that it is feasible to use response surface models to titrate propofol and remifentanil effect-site concentration, although this does not necessarily lead to comparable haemodynamic and electroencephalographic conditions. Their study identified combinations of effect-site propofol and remifentanil concentrations resulting in optimal clinical effects on many desired endpoints of a balanced anesthesia. In all studied groups, a variable number of patients needed treatment for hypotension during the non-steady state induction phase, suggesting that covariates other than the different combinations of propofol and remifentanil concentrations should be explored to optimize the haemodynamic control during anesthesia.

Different opioids have very different pharmacokinetic profiles, and so when they are used in combination with a hypnotic agent, they will affect the rate at which consciousness is regained when the anaesthetic administration ceases. The rate at which a patient will regain consciousness thus depends on the choice of agents, the respective doses, the sensitivity of the patient to the effects of the agents and in the case of agents whose elimination is context-sensitive, the duration of infusions of the agents used. If two agents are used in combination, then the fastest possible recovery can be achieved if a higher dose of the agent with the quickest "offset" is used in combination with a lower dose of the "slower" agent.

The pharmacodynamic interactions of propofol and remifentanil with regard to control of spontaneous breathing have also been studied.[211] LaPierre et al. explored remifentanil-propofol combinations that lead to a loss of response to esophageal instrumentation, a loss of responsiveness, and/or an onset of ventilatory depression requiring intervention.[174] They found that the combinations that allowed esophageal instrumentation and avoided intolerable ventilatory depression and/or loss of responsiveness primarily clustered around remifentanil-propofol effect-site concentrations ranging from 0.8 to 1.6 ng/ml and 1.5 to 2.7 µg/ml, respectively. However, blocking the response to esophageal instrumentation and avoiding both intolerable ventilatory depression and/or a loss of responsiveness is difficult. It may be necessary to accept some discomfort and blunt, rather than block, the response to esophageal instrumentation to consistently avoid intolerable ventilatory depression and/or loss of responsiveness.

Recently, our group studied the pharmacodynamic interaction between remifentanil (using the Eleveld remifentanil model) and dexmedetomidine (using the Hannivoort-Colin model) in 30 age- and sex- stratified healthy volunteers.[212] Drug effects were measured using binary (yes/no) endpoints and using the electroencephalogram derived 'Patient State index' (PSI, Masimo, Irvine,

CA, USA). We found that low dexmedetomidine concentrations (EC50 of 0.49 ng/ml) are required to induce sedation as measured by Patient State Index. Sensitivity to dexmedetomidine increases with age. Despite falling asleep, the majority of subjects remained arousable by calling the subject's name, "shake and shout", or a trapezius squeeze, even when reaching supra-clinical concentrations. Adding remifentanil does not alter the likelihood of response to graded stimuli. The cerebral drug effect as measured by the Patient State Index, was best described by the Hierarchical interaction model with an estimated dexmedetomidine EC50 of 0.49 ng/ml and remifentanil EC50 of 1.6 ng/ml.

4

—

Practical aspects

Manual infusion regimens

In this section some standardised manual infusion regimens will be described to assist those who do not have access to TCI technology, or who prefer, for whatever reason, to use manually controlled infusions. With these regimens it is possible to achieve steady state plasma concentrations quite quickly. The concentrations achieved will not be suitable for all patients, but should instead be used as a starting point from which infusion rates are adjusted according to the needs of the individual patient. Titrating to effect can be more precisely and rapidly performed with TCI systems, whereas the best the anaesthetist can do when titrating a manually controlled infusion is to have an educated guess at the sizes of boluses or infusion rate changes that need to be made to sufficiently increase or decrease the plasma and effect-site concentration of an anaesthetic drug.

PROPOFOL

A commonly used scheme is that proposed by Roberts and colleagues,[213] which gives a fairly close approximation to a steady state concentration of 3 μg/ml. It should be remembered that Roberts and colleges administered 3 μg/kg of fentanyl before starting the propofol infusion, and then mechanically ventilated the lungs of their patients with 67% N_2O. The infusion scheme involves an initial bolus of 1 mg/kg at induction followed by 10 mg/kg/hr for 10 minutes, then 8 mg/kg/hr for 10 minutes and finally 6 mg/kg/hr. Figure 3, panel D shows the plasma and effect-site concentrations during the first 60 minutes, as estimated by the Eleveld model.[79] Figure 3, panel C shows that if the initial bolus of 1 mg/ kg is omitted, then the estimated concentrations during the first 30 minutes will be substantially lower.

Because the kinetics of propofol are generally linear – for example if the size of the initial bolus and subsequent infusion rates are doubled the plasma concentration achieved will also be doubled. Thus an anaesthetist wishing to adjust the Robert infusion regime to achieve a different target concentration should make a proportional adjustment to the infusion rates. As mentioned earlier, while this sort of regimen can easily be used to achieve (close to) steady state plasma concentrations, it is not easy to accurately achieve different magnitudes of proportional change to the target concentration over time. Rapid changes in plasma concentration can only be achieved by boluses. A simple rule of thumb is that a 0.25 mg/kg bolus given to a healthy adult patient will temporarily increase the plasma propofol concentration by 3 µg/ml.

REMIFENTANIL

For induction of anaesthesia, a commonly used regimen is to give an infusion of 0.5 µg/kg/min for 3 minutes, followed by an infusion of 0.25 µg/kg/min. With this regimen steady state plasma concentrations result after about 8 minutes (approximately 6 ng/ml in younger patients, and 9 ng/ml in elderly patients – see Figure 9).

As can be inferred from Figure 9, it takes a few minutes before therapeutic effect-site concentrations will be achieved with this regimen. If a more rapid onset of action is desired then a bolus dose can be given, but to avoid adverse events, it should always be given slowly. One approach is to administer the bolus "on top of" the initial infusion rate over 1 minute. Using the regimens described above, an anaesthetist wishing to administer a careful bolus may set the pump to deliver an infusion at 1 µg/kg/min for 1 minute, then reduce the rate to 0.5 µg/kg/min for a further 2 minutes before making further reductions in infusion rate. This regimen will result in an almost step-wise increase in plasma concentration to ~6 ng/ml. Fit, young patients will usually tolerate this regimen very well. The bolus dose should be halved in elderly patients, and omitted in those who are very frail or unwell. In fit young patients maintenance infusion rates of between 0.12 and 0.5 µg/kg/min usually suffice (rates higher than that are rarely needed). Once again these rates should be reduced in the elderly (typically infusion rates between 0.08 and 0.25 µg/kg/min are sufficient).

SUFENTANIL

Glass et al. have recommended manual infusion schemes for sufentanil.[214] For sedation or analgesia, a loading dose of between 0.1 and 0.5 µg/kg, followed by an infusion of 0.005 – 0.01 µg/kg/min is recommended and should generate a plasma concentration of approximately 0.2 ng/ml. For general anaesthesia Glass recommend a loading dose of 1 – 5 µg/kg followed by an infusion at 0.01 –

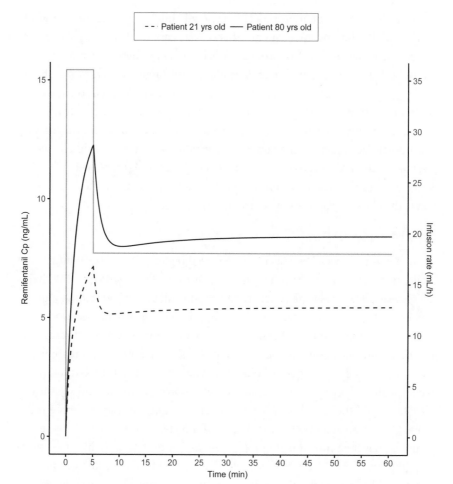

Figure 9: Predicted remifentanil plasma concentration and infusion rates during weight adjusted manual infusion (0.5 µg/kg/min for the first 5 minutes, followed by 0.25 µg/kg/min) in two female patients who both weigh 60 kg (height 165 cm) but have different ages (21 versus 80 years old). Note that in the older patient the same weight-adjusted infusion scheme resulted in far higher plasma concentrations than in the younger patient. Remifentanil concentration in syringe = 50 µg/ml

0.05 µg/kg/min. After an initial overshoot this regimen should generate plasma concentrations between 0.6 and 3 ng/ml. However, clinical experience shows that concentration between 0.1 and 0.4 ng/ml are sufficient for most operations, and that higher concentrations are only required during cardiac surgery.

KETAMINE

When ketamine is the sole agent used for induction of anaesthesia, bolus doses of between 1 and 2 mg/kg are required. A bolus dose of 2 mg/kg will typically produce 10 – 15 minutes of anaesthesia. For maintenance, infusion rates of 1 – 2 mg/kg/hr are needed. A bolus dose of 2 mg/kg followed by an infusion at 2 mg/kg/hr will result in concentrations of approximately 800 ng/ml (Domino model).

When ketamine is being used as an adjunct to another hypnotic agent, lower doses are required. Typical doses recommended for an anti-hyperalgesic effect are an infusion at 0.5 mg/kg/hr. If no bolus is given, plasma concentrations will increase for several hours. After 60 minutes, several hours before steady state is reached, the estimate plasma concentration will be 170 ng/ml (Domino model).

The above dosage schemes refer to racemic ketamine formulations. For esketamine, doses and infusion rates should be halved.

Target-controlled infusions

CHOICE OF PROPOFOL MODEL

Generally, it is advisable that anaesthetists choose one model, understand it and learn how to use it. Ideally, for the sake of safety, it is recommended that each department should choose and activate only one model per drug.[215] Anaesthetists with experience of administering propofol by TCI to children will have used either the Paedfusor or Kataria models in plasma targeting mode when using the second generation of TCI pumps. Most anaesthetists already familiar with TCI administration of propofol in adults, will have used a system programmed with the Schnider or Marsh model. In general, the Schnider model should always be used in effect-site targeting mode. Most anaesthetists currently using the Marsh model use it in plasma targeting mode, although some use it in effect-site mode, using a 'modified Marsh' model (i.e. one with a keo of 1.26 min⁻¹). As this "modified Marsh model" has only historical value, we strongly recommend that it is no longer used. For most healthy, young and middle-aged adults, the differences in dose administered between effect-site targeted Schnider and plasma targeted Marsh will be small. For the same target concentration, the dose administered in the initial 10 minutes will be somewhat smaller with the former, but thereafter the infusion rates will be rather similar. For very tall, thin patients, maintenance infusion rates will be higher with the Schnider model.[70] On the other hand, experienced users will know that for a given target concentration, in elderly patients the infusion rates will be lower for the Schnider model than the Marsh model.

The availability of different adult and paediatric propofol models, with different modes (plasma versus effect-site targeting) and sometimes even different methods of implementing effect-site targeting, is less than ideal.[70] It has resulted in endless discussions about which model is superior, which is seen by some as an unnecessary distraction. More importantly, when several options are available to the clinician, this can cause confusion and increase the chances of errors.[215] We believe that if the available general purpose models are implemented in TCI pumps, this will improve safety. It is anticipated that by the end of 2019 the Eleveld model will be available in several infusion pumps. We hope that this model will be widely adopted into clinical practice, and that it will be used in effect-site targeting mode. One of the advantages of the Eleveld model is that it takes into account the presence (or absence) of opioids.

DIFFERENCES BETWEEN ELEVELD, SCHNIDER AND MARSH MODELS

The development and details of the different models has been discussed earlier. What the clinician needs to know is how the doses and infusion rates differ between the models, to help inform their choice of model and of target concentration. The differences between doses delivered will of course depend on the patient characteristics. Figure 10 illustrates the influence of choice of model on cumulative propofol dose for a representative patient, a 170cm tall man, whose weight is 75 kg and age 45. It shows the cumulative volume of 1% propofol infused with a target concentration of 3 µg/ml with the Marsh (plasma targeting), Schnider (*effect-site* targeting; fixed keo and fixed TTPE implementations) and Eleveld (*effect-site* targeting) models. As can be seen in the figure, for a patient with the above-mentioned characteristics, the initial dose administered by the Eleveld model (effect-site targeting mode) is significantly larger than that administered with the Marsh model (plasma targeting mode) and the Schnider model (effect-site targeting mode). After the first few minutes the infusion rates of the Eleveld model and Marsh model are somewhat similar, so that the difference in cumulative doses remains roughly the same. The infusion rates of the Eleveld model are higher than those of the Schnider model, which is why there is a gradual divergence in the cumulative doses with the Eleveld and Schnider models. In this patient, the cumulative dose administered with the two implementations of the Schnider model is the same at all time points. This is not the case at the extremes of height and weight.[70]

Those colleagues more familiar with the Schnider model will notice that, generally, for the same target concentrations, the initial bolus dose size will be significantly greater, and loss of consciousness more rapid, with the Eleveld

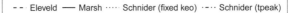

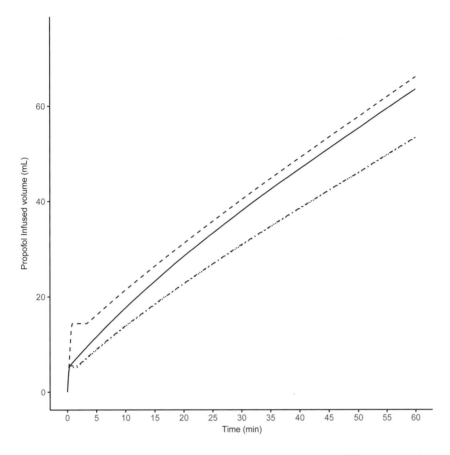

Figure 10: Comparison of the cumulative dose of propofol 1 % infused when a TCI system uses the March model in plasma mode, the Schnider model with fixed ke0 in effect-site mode, the Schnider model with fixed tpeak in effect-site mode and the Eleveld model in effect-site mode at a target concentration of 3 μg/ml. Patient is male, 45 years, height 170 cm, weight 75 kg.

model, than with the Schnider model. Those more familiar with the Marsh model will notice that for the same target concentrations the initial doses will also be larger than those of the Marsh model in plasma mode, but similar to those administered with the modified Marsh model in effect-site targeting mode.

In older patients, the Eleveld will administer similar doses to the Schnider model, but less than the Marsh model, whereas in children the doses will be similar to those of the Paedfusor and Kataria models. Finally, in obese patients, the Eleveld will administer propofol doses intermediate between that of the Marsh model (when the actual weight is programmed in the pump) and the Schnider model.

As propofol doses differ between models for the same target concentration, it is recommended that anaesthetists understand not only the differences between models, but also have a good idea of which target concentrations are appropriate for each model. If this advice is not followed, and users apply the same target concentrations for the Eleveld model as they do for the Marsh model then initial doses will be higher than expected, whereas subsequent infusion rates will be similar to what they expect. If users apply the same initial target concentrations for the Eleveld model as they do for the Schnider model then initial doses will be **much** higher than expected, and subsequent infusion rates will also be faster than what they are used to.

Suggested ranges of target concentrations will be given in the following sections.

SUGGESTED TARGET CONCENTRATIONS FOR PROPOFOL SEDATION

With the use of the Marsh or Schnider model, most patients will experience anxiolysis with target concentrations in the range of 0.8 – 1.2 µg/ml. The range of target concentrations required for sedation is broader, being approximately 0.8 – 2.0 µg/ml. Titration to effect is almost always needed, as is adjustment for the age and health of the patient. Younger and more anxious patients tend to need higher target concentrations, whereas sicker, elderly patients need lower concentrations (bear in mind that at target concentrations of 2.0 µg/ml some elderly patients will lose consciousness). When a patient has already received an opioid it is wise to select a somewhat lower initial target propofol concentration.

When using the Eleveld model for propofol the age-based model-predicted target concentrations can be used as a guide. In fact, as can be seen from Figure 8, for mild to moderate sedation (BIS of 84), for most adult patients an effect-site concentration of approximately 1.0 µg/ml should be sufficient. For an 80 year old patient approximately 0.7 µg/ml is needed on average.

INDUCTION AND MAINTENANCE OF PROPOFOL-BASED ANAESTHESIA

General advice

No single regimen, concentration or drug combination applies to all patients. Target concentrations should be individually determined based on patient characteristics (health status, anxiety etc), the model chosen, and whether or not other drugs have been administered. There is wide variability in individual patient pharmacokinetics and pharmacodynamics, and pharmacokinetic and dynamic interactions between co-administered drugs can be strong and significant. As with inhalational anaesthesia clinical judgement is always required, and the doses of drugs used should be titrated according to the clinical response of the patient.

When consciousness is lost, and again during manipulation of the airway (tracheal intubation or laryngeal mask insertion) it is advisable to take note of the estimated effect-site propofol concentration to give further "calibration points" for the patient's sensitivity to propofol. For example if the blood pressure and heart rate do not change during tracheal intubation then it is safe to assume that the effect-site concentration at that time was adequate for a noxious stimulus. During the operation the patient should be observed closely. The target concentration should be adjusted according to the clinical responses of the patient.

There are significant differences in pharmacokinetic and dynamics of propofol in the elderly compared with younger patients. The Schnider and Eleveld model adjust model parameters to take account of age-related pharmacokinetic differences, resulting in lower doses for the same target concentration than in younger patients. On the other hand, the Marsh model makes no such allowances for age. Accordingly, when the Marsh model is used, the anaesthetist must select lower target concentrations to make allowance for the kinetic and dynamic differences.

Remember too that the propofol requirements will also be influenced by the co-administration of other agents that influence depth of anaesthesia such as ketamine, opioids, nitrous oxide and benzodiazepines.

When neuromuscular blocking agents are used, extra caution should be followed, and a processed EEG monitor should ideally be used (as recommended by recently published guidelines[215]).

Towards the end of the case, as the intensity of the surgical stimulus reduces, the target concentrations can be gradually reduced to promote a more rapid recovery from anaesthesia. Generally the infusion can be stopped once the final sutures or dressings are applied. Stopping the infusion is best done by reducing the target concentration to zero, so that the pump continues to show the estimated plasma and effect-site concentrations.

When using TCI it is always advisable to look at the infusion rate intermittently, to confirm that it is roughly consistent with what is expected. This is particularly valuable when more than one drug is used (it can help alert the user to a 'syringe swap error') or when a new or unfamiliar model is in use.

The following model-specific advice should only be used as a guide. The recommendations are based on a combination of our clinical experience, and published studies on the ranges target concentrations at loss and return of consciousness.

As a general rule in fragile patients, it is always advised to start with a lower target, watch the effect at time to peak effect and, if required, increase the target in small steps.

Marsh Model

If a relatively rapid induction of anaesthesia is required, initial plasma propofol target concentrations of 4–6 µg/ml are typically used in healthy young or middle-aged patients. Occasionally, fit young patients who are very anxious, have not received a sedative premedication and/or have not yet received any opioids, may require even higher target concentrations for loss of consciousness (6 –8 µg/ml). In these patients it is probably acceptable to start at target concentrations of 6 µg/ml, and then adjust the target upwards every 30 sec as required.

In older, frail or unwell patients, lower starting concentrations are recommended (2 – 4.0 µg/ml), with slow target concentration increases in increments of 0.5 µg/ml as needed. In patients with cardiac compromise, it is wise to "start low and go slow". By this we mean begin at a target concentration of 1 – 1.5 µg/ml, and only make increments of 0.5 µg/ml after intervals of 2 – 3 .

When the modified Marsh model is used in effect-site targeting mode, then for the same target concentration, initial doses will be far higher. Effect-site targeting is probably unwise in the elderly and/or unwell, and in younger and more healthy patients, it is wise to choose a conservative initial target concentration (e.g. at the lower end of the ranges mentioned below).

After loss of consciousness and endotracheal intubation, target concentrations are usually reduced. Larger decreases may be needed if there is a long interval between induction of anaesthesia and the first skin incision (something familiar to most readers). During maintenance of anaesthesia, target concentrations of 3.0 – 6.0 µg/ml (without opioids) or 2.5–4.0 µg/ml (with opioids) are typical. Occasionally, when opioids are in use, target concentrations of 1.5 – 2.0 µg/ml are sufficient for frail elderly patients.

Schnider model

For the Schnider model, the general advice above should be followed. This model should always be used in effect-site targeting mode.

The lower panel of Figure 8 shows the influence of age on the EC_{50} required for loss of consciousness (responsiveness), as determined in Schnider's original studies. It should be borne in mind that for laryngoscopy, intubation and surgery, somewhat higher effect-site concentrations will be needed (depending on the co-administered opioid doses). For the choice of target concentrations, our advice is therefore to use similar or slightly higher target concentrations than those recommended above for the Marsh model for both induction and maintenance. Just as with the Marsh model, anaesthetists commonly use lower target concentrations during maintenance of anaesthesia than during induction and laryngoscopy.[179]

Eleveld model

We believe that the Eleveld model should always be used in effect-site targeting mode. Users should note however, that when used in this mode, the initial doses and infusion rates may be different to those for the same target concentrations with other models, with the nature and direction of the differences depending on the age and other patient characteristics.

As has been mentioned, the PK part of the Eleveld model adjusts infusion rates according to age, so that for a given target concentration, lower propofol doses are administered. A unique feature of the combined PK/PD model is that the PD component enables the calculation of the estimated effect-site target concentration necessary to achieve a given percentage decline in the BIS value, for a given patient. In the model, the baseline BIS is 94. We refer to the effect-site concentration necessary for an x% decline from this baseline, as the ECx. This 'EC50' is strongly dependent on age (see Figure 8, upper panel).

Given that BIS values of around 50 are recommended for induction of anaesthesia, a reasonable initial choice is the EC50 – the effect-site concentration likely to be associated with a BIS of 47 for a patient of that age. This approach takes account of the pharmacokinetic differences in patients (influence of age and other co-variates on the doses required to achieve a given concentration) as well as on the pharmacodynamic differences (influence of age on the concentration needed for a given clinical effect). As can be seen in Figure 8, the effect of age on the EC50 is quite strong. Whereas for an 90 year old patient the EC50 is 2.17 µg/ml, for an 18 year patient it is 3.43 µg/ml.

With the Eleveld model the EC50 for all adults will be much lower than the usual intial target concentrations selected for the Marsh and Schnider model. Anaesthetists changing from using other models to using the Eleveld are urged to keep this in mind, as selection of target concentrations in the familiar 4 – 6 µg/ml range will likely result in very large, potentially harmful doses.

As always, with use of the Eleveld model, other factors should be taken into consideration, such as the nature of the procedure, and the fitness of the patient. Whereas the Eleveld model does alter the PK parameters when other drugs are administered – to adjust for pharmacokinetic interactions – the PD component cannot yet take into account pharmacodynamics interactions. Changes to the target concentrations may be necessary to account for when other drugs are administered that may cause pharmacodynamic interactions with propofol.

Advice for the complete TIVA novice

Anaesthetists wishing to use intravenous maintenance of anaesthesia for the first time should ideally first observe a colleague practising TIVA, and ideally also attend a practical workshop, such as the workshops held at one of the several national and international intravenous anaesthesia societies. They should then choose their first cases carefully, and not jump directly in the "deep end." For example, it is best not to start with a case during which unexpected movements are disastrous (e.g. a vitrectomy).

As with all clinical skills, there are many different ways of achieving the same goal. The advice that follows should be followed in a general sense, bearing in mind that all patients are different, doses should always be titrated to clinical effect, and of course there are remarkable differences in practice between different hospitals and different countries. Please do not apply the examples given here as fixed recipes!

Our personal opinion, concordant with the UK TIVA guidelines, is that for the novice a deeper level of knowledge is needed to manual TIVA, than for TCI.[215] We thus recommend that novices start straight off with TCI propofol, and use the system as they might use a vapouriser (e.g. titrate to effect). A safe way to acquire some basic clinical skills in intravenous anaesthesia is to start by using propofol TCI for procedural sedation or during surgical procedures performed under local or regional anaesthesia. Start at an initial target of 0.5 µg/ml (ideally using Eleveld in effect-site mode, but otherwise the Marsh model in plasma mode, or the Schnider model in effect-site mode), then wait and observe the clinical effect for a few minutes (ideally until time to peak effect for every step as shown in Figure 4. After that adjust the target concentration in small steps (0.1 – 0.2 µg/ml increments or decrements), observing the patient closely between steps. Remember that the dose or target concentration required will change if other drugs are used, and as the intensity of any noxious stimulus changes. If no TCI system is available, try administering 10 – 20 mg bolus, and use an infusion rate of the order of 3 mg/kg/hr.

When progressing on to use TIVA for the first time for general anaesthesia we would recommend starting with a minor surgical case in a fit patient aged 20 – 40. One option is to choose a case for which spontaneous ventilation via a laryngeal mask airway (LMA) is feasible, and for which local or regional anaesthesia is possible. There are many such cases; examples include operations for ingrown toenails, tendon or nerve repairs, knee arthroscopies, varicose veins stripping. Use a propofol TCI system if available, and ideally use the Eleveld model in effect-site mode. If no TCI pump is available, use an infusion pump that will allow the user to enter the infusion rate in mg/kg/hr, to enable the user to administer a variant of the Roberts regimen. If a monitor of anaesthetic depth is available then it should be used for further reassurance, and the electrodes applied for induction of anaesthesia. Before starting the propofol infusion, inject 2 – 3 ml of 1% lidocaine to attenuate any pain at the start of the propofol infusion. Two minutes before starting the propofol administer a modest intravenous dose of fentanyl or alfentanil (eg. 1 µg/kg fentanyl, or 10 µg/kg alfentanil). If using a TCI system, with the Eleveld model, use a chart such as that in Figure 8 to select an initial target that should generate a BIS of around 50. A general rule of thumb would be to select an initial target 3.5 µg/ml in young adults, 2.0 µg/ml in the very old, and somewhere in between for middle-aged adults. If the Eleveld model is not available, select an initial target concentration of 4 µg/ml for the Marsh model (plasma mode) or Schnider model (effect-site mode).

Once this initial target concentration has been achieved, assess the conscious state of the patient continuously, and increase the target concentration in steps of 0.5 µg/ml until the patient no longer responds to voice and the eyelash reflex is lost. Observe the effect-site concentration at loss of consciousness. Once the patient's jaw is sufficiently relaxed, attempt LMA insertion. If the jaw is not relaxed, or the patient resists LMA insertion, wait a little longer, and increase the target concentration if necessary.

Once the LMA has been inserted, the effect-site propofol concentration can usually be reduced to a slightly lower level than was present during LMA insertion. Assist ventilation manually until spontaneous ventilation returns, using 30 – 40% O_2 in air (or 60 – 70% N_2O/30 – 40% O_2 mix). If feasible perform a nerve or field local anaesthetic block. If propofol is used without an opioid, N_2O or regional block then higher doses/target concentrations will be required.

"Invite" the surgeon to start the operation once you are confident the patient is adequately anaesthetised and cardiovascular parameters are stable. If the patient becomes tachypnoeic, or tachycardic, increase the target propofol concentration, and consider administering another modest dose of fentanyl or alfentanil. If the blood pressure is low, and the patient remains apnoeic for longer than expected, it may be necessary to reduce the target propofol concentration.

When the surgeon is starting to close the wound, reduce the target propofol concentration by ~25%; once the suture is in place, switch off the infusion and the nitrous oxide, and observe the rapid and clear-headed recovery of the patient!

Starting with spontaneously breathing, non-paralysed patients add extra layers of safety, since it enables the anaesthetist to also titrate drug doses according to ventilatory responses, while giving the reassurance that if anaesthesia is inadequate, the patient will be able to move, or even leave the room!

Eventually, with further experience and confidence, more challenging cases can be attempted, including ones where muscle relaxation is required. For long cases, or any case where endotracheal intubation is needed, propofol/remifentanil is a very nice combination. The remifentanil will reduce the propofol dose requirements, and will inhibit movement in response to pain, or coughing or bucking on an endotracheal tube. Mostly, a target concentration of >4 ng/ml will prevent movement or coughing. Bear in mind however, that it is difficult to maintain spontaneous ventilation whilst a patient receives remifentanil and propofol, so that mechanical ventilation will almost certainly be required, although this is quite easily achieved via a LMA in many patients without muscle relaxants.

Target-controlled infusions of opioids

Target-controlled infusions of opioids are widely used. Of the currently available open TCI infusion pumps, all are programmed to allow TCI administration of remifentanil. Some also have models loaded for one or more of sufentanil, alfentanil and fentanyl.

Effect-site targeting seems to us to be a logical choice. If blood targeting is used and rapid onset of analgesia is required, then the plasma concentration should initially be set to a level higher than the likely therapeutic effect-site concentration. After induction of anaesthesia, the target concentrations should be adjusted according to the clinical responses of the patient. Patient movement, and increases in heart rate and blood pressure, in response to an increase in the intensity of noxious stimulus are most logically treated by increases in the level of analgesia.

ADDED VALUE OF TCI REMIFENTANIL (VERSUS MANUAL ADMINISTRATION)

When fixed rate remifentanil infusions are used steady-state concentrations are reached far sooner than with most other anaesthetic drugs (after an infusion duration of about 15 minutes the plasma concentrations reach a plateau). More importantly, the decline in remifentanil concentration after an infusion is stopped is far more predictable than the decline found with other drugs. Regardless of the duration of the infusion the context-sensitive half-time (the time after the infusion is stopped that it takes for the plasma concentration to fall by 50%) remains of the order of 4 minutes. This context-insensitivity is in stark contrast with most other anaesthetic agents whose context-sensitive half-times increase with the duration of the infusion.[90][216]

These beneficial pharmacokinetic properties of remifentanil have led many to question the need for TCI remifentanil systems. Many anaesthetists administer manually controlled remifentanil infusions using fairly simple regimens in which the infusion rate is calculated only on the basis of the weight of the patient. While weight-adjusted infusion regimens work well for young healthy patients they can give far higher plasma concentrations than expected in elderly or unwell patients. Minto found that the pharmacokinetics of remifentanil are affected by age, gender and height, in addition to weight. The simulation in Figure 9 uses the Minto model to show the predicted plasma concentrations that would arise from the same infusion profile in two female patients both weighing 60 kg, but with different heights and weights. In both remifentanil is infused at 0.5 μg/kg/min for 5 min and thereafter at 0.25μg/kg/min. After 15 min the plasma concentration in the younger, taller patient is approximately 5 ng/ml, whereas in the older, shorter patient the plasma concentration is about 8 ng/ml. Given that the elderly patient is likely to also have greater (pharmacodynamic) sensitivity to the effects of remifentanil, this concentration is likely to result in clinical effects at least twice as great as those in the younger patient, with the potential for serious adverse effects.

On the other side of the age spectrum – in children – the opposite problem occurs, as significantly higher infusion rates are needed to achieve the same plasma concentrations as in adults. A group with even more complex changes in pharmacokinetics is the group of obese adults, in whom model parameters do not scale linearly with total body mass, and in whom clearance parameters probably scale better allometrically with size.[60][64]

Thus, while manual infusion regimens are probably satisfactory in younger, fitter patients in whom excessive concentrations are better tolerated, in obese adults, in the elderly and unwell, and in children, more precise administration regimens are required.

It would be time-consuming and complicated for an anaesthetist to calculate infusion rates based on age, weight, height, and gender, using non-linear scaling methods. The most precise control of remifentanil concentrations can be achieved with a TCI system that is programmed with a sophisticated model that works well in that population. Whereas the Minto model works well in adults of normal weight, and also makes appropriate adjustments in the elderly, it is not validated for use in children and has problems when used in the obese (see later explanation of the problems of the James equation). When the Kim and Eleveld remifentanil models are implemented in TCI pumps, we believe that they will help anaesthetists to optimize remifentanil administration. The data set used to develop the Eleveld model did not contain data from obese patients, but does employ allometric size scaling, and makes appropriate adjustments to its model parameters in the elderly and in children.[64] The Kim model was developed using data sets from obese and non-obese adults, and so will facilitate accurate titration of remifentanil in obese and non-obese adults, but is not suitable for use in children.[86]

EFFECT-SITE TARGETED OPIOID INFUSIONS

Effect-site targeted TCI administration of opioids is possible for drugs for which k_{eo} values have been calculated or for which the TTPE is known; and when stepwise changes in effect-site opioid concentrations are required or desirable, effect-site targeting may be useful. There are a few problems with effect-site targeting of opioids. The first is that there have been few combined pharmacokinetic-dynamic studies. For most of the opioids, the k_{eo} values that have been published have been determined from pure pharmacodynamic studies in which the measure of clinical effect was one or more of the parameters derived from the spontaneous EEG (such as SEF and MF). These parameters have not been conclusively shown to correlate with clinical indicators of analgesia.

For remifentanil, Minto and colleagues did perform a formal combined pharmacokinetic and dynamic study. The k_{eo} that they derived is adjusted for age as follows: $k_{eo} = 0.595 - 0.007 \times (age - 40)$.[55] For alfentanil a k_{eo} value of 0.77 min^{-1} is sometimes used to calculate effect-site concentrations. This value, also used by Maitre and colleagues in their study of the pharmacokinetics of alfentanil,[97] was determined from a study performed by Scott et al.[217] For sufentanil, the k_{eo} value of 0.119 min^{-1} calculated by Scott and colleagues[218] is sometimes used with the Gepts model to calculate effect-site concentrations.

When a k_{eo} is used during plasma concentration targeted infusions to simply estimate the effect-site concentration, errors are less clinically significant. As mentioned earlier, during effect-site targeted infusions the choice of k_{eo} is more critical, because it will significantly affect the rate of infusion of drug after a change in target concentration. Given that TTPE values for sufentanil and alfentanil have been published (5.4 and 1.4 min respectively),[219] it is probably better to use a TTPE method to calculate individualised k_{eo} values when effect-site targeted infusions of sufentanil and alfentanil are administered.

So, is effect-site targeting really necessary for the opiates? In the case of remifentanil, the case for effect-site targeting is less compelling, because simulations show that when using a plasma targeted infusion, equilibration between plasma and effect-site concentrations is virtually complete within 5 minutes. With plasma concentration targeting, rapid rises in effect-site concentration can be achieved by brief periods of overshoot. When effect-site targeting is used, the overshoot is of course calculated and controlled automatically. Because the plasma concentration of remifentanil falls so rapidly after an infusion stops, an effect-site targeted remifentanil infusion system is able to choose very high target plasma concentrations, and in doing so to achieve almost step-wise increases in estimated effect-site concentrations. Although the overshoot will only be temporary it is worth bearing in mind, or placing a limit of the degree of overshoot. If the Minto model is used for effect-site targeting, and the overshoot is not limited, an initial effect-site target of 6 ng/ml will require a peak plasma concentration of 17 ng/ml, a level that may be associated with adverse effects such as chest wall rigidity and bradycardia in compromised patients.

The argument is somewhat stronger for opioids that do not equilibrate as rapidly with the effect-site, such as sufentanil. With these drugs, effect-site targeting will hasten the onset of clinical effect. It is difficult to find compelling reasons for using effect-site targeted (or even plasma concentration targeted) infusions of opioids such as morphine and fentanyl that accumulate because of slow metabolism and/or large volumes of distribution.

CHOICE OF INITIAL TARGET CONCENTRATIONS

It should be remembered that as with the hypnotics, no firm recommendations can be made for target concentrations for the opioids, since pharmacokinetic and pharmacodynamic differences between patients make it essential to titrate the target concentration according to the intensity of the surgical stimulus and of course the patient response. Titration to effect-based on clinical signs is always required. At present clinicians mostly judge the adequacy of the nociception-antinociception balance on the basis of clinical signs such as heart rate, blood pressure and movement in response to pain.

The therapeutic concentrations for the commonly used opioids have already been mentioned in the Pharmacodynamics section (pages 48 and 49), and so will only be briefly re-visited here with an emphasis on more practical aspects.

If remifentanil is used, effect-site concentrations of the order of 4 – 6 ng/ml are required for adequate analgesia during laryngoscopy and tracheal intubation. Slightly lower concentrations are necessary for laryngeal mask airway insertion. During very painful operations such as laparotomy, concentrations of

6 – 8 ng/ml are usually necessary, whereas during cardiac surgery concentrations of the order of 10 – 12 ng/ml may be needed.

For alfentanil, target concentrations of approximately 80 – 100 ng/ml are required for laryngoscopy and other very painful procedures such as peritoneal incision. During less painful procedures target concentrations of 40 – 80 ng/ml are common, whereas during cardiac surgery, where the hypnotic-sparing effect of the opioids will enhance cardio-stability, target concentrations in the range 120 – 200 ng/ml are commonly used.

Sufentanil is a good alternative for longer operations, as it is cheaper, and has a PK profile reasonably well suited for TCI administration. For TCI administration of sufentanil, target concentrations of 0.3 ng/ml are commonly used. This results in an initial bolus of 15 – 20 µg. For cardiac surgery target concentrations of up to 1.0 ng/ml are used. It is wise to generally use effect-site targeting with sufentanil as the plasma and effect-site concentrations equilibrate rather slowly. Even with the latter it should be noticed that it will take a few minutes for the effect-site concentration to reach its target value, and is advisable to the sufentanil infusion 2 – 3 minutes before inducing anaesthesia with propofol (regardless of whether the propofol is administered by manual bolus or infusion or TCI). If there is a need for a more rapid attainment of adequate effect-site concentrations, then a higher initial target concentration can be selected. It should be remembered that the kinetics of sufentanil are highly context-sensitive. After prolonged infusions, it can take more than an hour before plasma concentrations reduce to levels at which spontaneous breathing is likely (±0.1 ng/ml). For this reason it is best to stop the infusion (or reduce the target to zero) at least an hour before the end of the operation.

Target concentrations for fentanyl are commonly between 1 and 3 ng/ml.

WHICH DRUG INFUSION SHOULD BE STARTED FIRST

When propofol/remifentanil combinations are used, different groups have different ideas about which agent to start first at induction of anaesthesia. Much depends on the mode of administration. If the anaesthetist has opted for a manual infusion, and does not administer a bolus of remifentanil, then it takes several minutes before therapeutic concentrations are reached. In this case, it makes sense to start the remifentanil infusion 3 – 5 minutes before a hypnotic drug is being administered. An added advantage of starting the remifentanil first is that the patient will experience less discomfort from the propofol. However, if remifentanil is administered by TCI the picture is somewhat different, since the plasma and effect-site remifentanil concentrations will rise more rapidly, and therefore cross the thresholds at which respiratory depression and apnoea occur. If the remifentanil infusion is started first the patient is more likely to stop breathing before loss of consciousness, and if loss of consciousness occurs slowly, this may result in hypoxaemia while the airway is being secured, even if the patient was pre-oxygenated with 100% O_2. On some occasions it may be necessary to use bag and mask ventilation to improve oxygenation before consciousness is completely lost, and this may cause the patient distress. Arguments for starting the propofol infusion first, are that propofol has slower kinetics than that of remifentanil, and also equilibrates more slowly with the effect-site. Anecdotal reports also suggest that chest wall rigidity associated with high doses of remifentanil is less likely if propofol is given before the remifentanil infusion is started.

TIVA and TCI in obese patients

For most drugs used in clinical practice, whether by bolus or infusion or both, the doses and infusion rates recommended in the package inserts are calculated on a weight-adjusted basis. The problem with this is that most of the pharmacokinetic studies involving anaesthetic agents have only included healthy, non-obese patients, and very few have specifically studied the pharmacokinetic properties of these drugs in obese patients. While the recommended weight-adjusted doses apply to most patients, anaesthetists in clinical practice soon intuitively realise that they do not apply to obese, elderly or unwell patients, for whom a smaller dose will usually be given. For example, a patient who is 170 cm tall and weighs 140 kg does not usually need twice as much propofol to induce anaesthesia as a patient who has the same height but weighs only 70 kg. Conversely, two patients of similar weight, but with marked differences in height and age, do not require the same dose of remifentanil (Figure 9) to achieve the same plasma concentration.

The intuitive inclination of anaesthetists to reduce the weight-adjusted dose in the obese is supported by studies that have shown a good correlation between dose requirements and **lean body mass** for propofol,[220] thiopentone,[221] and atracurium.[222] A study by Egan and colleagues of remifentanil pharmacokinetics in obese and non-obese patients showed that if doses are calculated according to total body weight, then measured concentrations are significantly higher in obese patients.[88] Also the study showed that if compartment volumes are clearances are adjusted for lean body mass, then the pharmacokinetics among obese and non-obese patients are similar, leading the authors to conclude that dose regimens for remifentanil should be based on ideal body weight or lean body mass.

Models developed for TCI administration of drugs used in anaesthesia were mostly also developed from data from patients or volunteers that were fit, young, healthy, and of normal weight. When such models are used for TCI in obese patients, such extrapolation is generally associated with poor predictive performance.[70][79] Use of the Marsh or Schnider model for propofol administration is problematic for the patients with obesity grade II or worse (i.e. BMI > 35 kg/m^2). The two models present different practical problems – to be explained below – and so over time, anaesthetists developed practical ways of dealing with the short-comings of models not developed for the obese population. These pragmatic solutions, involving the user entering weight (and sometimes height and gender) values different to those of the patient, were an imperfect and fallible interim solution that enabled the skilled anaesthetist to safely administer propofol (and similarly remifentanil) by TCI to obese patients.

One of the aims of the development of general purpose models for propofol[57] and remifentanil[64][86] was to make it easier for anaesthestists to administer propofol and remifentanil safely and simply by TCI, without the need for making somewhat arbitrary adjustments to the demographic patient data during pump programming. Instead of LBM, the Eleveld general purpose models for propofol and remifentanil both use fat-free mass (FFM) based on the Al-Sallami formula[223] which is a much better size descriptor for broadly applied PK models (from neonates to obese adults). With the use of these models and size descriptors, the user should enter the correct patient demographic details (no fancy things, just actual weight, age, height, gender), and leave it to the software of the pump to adjust the necessary infusion rates. We hope that these models will soon be well-accepted and implemented in practise – not because we want to promote our own models, but because we believe that it will benefit patients. If this goal is realised then the discussion below will be irrelevant.

In the Marsh model, all volumes scale linearly with weight, meaning that induction doses will be very large if the actual weight is used (in fact most pumps will not allow input of a weight >150kg). Anaesthetists experienced in intravenous anaesthesia will tend to input into the pump a lower value than the measured total body weight. One strategy is to have an arbitrary maximum weight, and if the patient weighs more than that, input that maximum value. It is important to remember, of course, that the maximum value used should depend on the height of the patient. Another strategy is to estimate the patient's ideal body weight (IBW) and then to use a figure somewhere between the ideal weight and the measured total body weight. A commonly used method of calculating IBW is by using the following formulae [224]:

Males: Ideal body weight (kg) = 49.9 + 0.89 × (height in cm – 152.4)
Females: Ideal body weight (kg) = 45.4 + 0.89 × (height in cm – 152.4)

A simpler method is the following 'rule of thumb':

Males: IBW (kg) = Height (cm) – 100
Females: IBW (kg) = Height (cm) – 105

Given the knowledge that use of the IBW during Marsh-based propofol TCI will result in a reasonable induction bolus, but inadequate maintenance rates, many anaesthetists opt for a pragmatic adjusted weight, as first suggested by Servin,[71] and implemented by others[225]:

Adjusted weight = IBW + [(total weight – IBW) × 0.4]

The Schnider model for propofol, and the Minto model for remifentanil, are more complex than the Marsh model and use age and **lean body mass** (LBM) as co-variables. These models require the user to enter the total body weight, height and gender, and then use these variables to calculate the lean body mass according to the following formulae[69]:

Males: LBM = 1.1 × weight – 128 × (weight/height)^2
Females: LBM = 1.07 × weight – 148 × (weight/height)^2

At first glance the use of LBM may seem like a sensible idea, and so it is for the non-obese population, for whom the equations give a reasonable approximation of the ideal body mass (Figure 7). The problem is that these equations do not apply to the (growing) population of extremely obese patients. As can be seen from the equations, for a given height, as the weight increases the LBM will increase, but a threshold will be reached beyond which the LBM will decrease (which is counter-intuitive) and eventually become negative (which is absurd)! This is illustrated in Figure 7.

   Automated infusion systems that seek to implement the Schnider and Minto models (and indeed any other model using LBM calculated with the James formula), should be programmed with a strategy for dealing with extremely obese patients. A system that blindly uses the LBM formulae given above for an extremely obese patient, is likely to administer far too little drug for remifentanil and too much for propofol (the difference arises from differences in how the LBM is used in the calculations of the model parameters). One approach is for the microprocessor to be programmed with absolute weight limits for total body weight, and to simply refuse to operate in TCI mode when those limits are exceeded. A more sophisticated approach is to program the pump to refuse to accept a figure for the patient weight if it exceeds the weight that generates the maximum LBM from the equations. In this situation the best compromise is probably to program the pump to suggest that the user inputs the body weight that generates the maximum LBM. For example if the patient is female and 150 cm tall but weighs more than 80 kg (see Figure 7), the pump should either refuse to operate in TCI mode, or suggest that the user inputs a value of 80 kg.

Both of the above-mentioned solutions have been used by different TCI pumps. Anaesthetists faced with a situation where the patient parameter exceeded the limits mentioned above, either simply inputted the maximum weight value the pump allowed, or entered 'male' for female patients, or entered a falsely elevated height value. As an alternative some entered an adjusted body weight, calculated as above, and found that the predictive performance of the system with these values was reasonable.[226]

Until the general purpose models are available and in general use, anaesthestists caring for obese patients should be aware of the problems involved, and the potential consequences of their chosen solution.

High risk patients (Elderly, unwell, or patients with limited cardiac reserve)

Caution should always be exercised with patients who are elderly, unwell or who have limited cardiovascular reserve. Because these patients have altered pharmacokinetics (volumes of distribution, and distribution and metabolic clearance rates are often reduced when compared with fitter, younger patients), equivalent doses calculated on the basis of body weight will often result in far higher plasma concentrations than would otherwise be expected. Moreover, for given plasma and effect-site concentrations the hypnotics and opiates tend to produce more profound pharmacodynamic effects in the elderly and unwell, because of greater receptor sensitivity. Not only do these patients lose consciousness at lower plasma and effect-site concentrations, they also will develop cardio-respiratory compromise at lower concentrations.

These differences in pharmacokinetics and pharmacodynamics in the elderly make it imperative to consider carefully the target concentrations to be used in these patients, and to titrate these according to effect even more carefully. Simpler models tend not to include age as a co-variate, and when these models are used to control a target-controlled infusion, then it is wise to use lower target concentrations for sedation and for induction and maintenance of anaesthesia.

In the very old and frail, or in patients with serious cardiac problems, it is best when inducing anaesthesia with TCI propofol, to start at very low target concentrations (e.g. 1.5 μg/ml) and to increase the target concentration in small steps (e.g. 0.5 μg/ml) every few minutes. With this approach, speed of induction is sacrificed in return for improved cardiovascular stability. In practise though, patients with cardiovascular compromise who are about to undergo cardiac surgery, typically have received a sedative pre-medication, and then a large dose of opioid during induction, and commonly lose consciousness at fairly low plasma and effect-site propofol concentrations.

In frail or unwell patients not undergoing cardiac surgery, improved cardiovascular stability can be achieved by using a combination of a moderately high dose of remifentanil (eg. an infusion rate of ~0.25 – 0.3 μg/kg/min or a target concentration of 6 – 8 ng/ml) with a lower dose of hypnotic (e.g. propofol infused at 3 – 5 mg/kg/hr or at a target concentration of 1.5 – 2.5 μg/ml). When these doses of remifentanil are used in these patients all airway reflexes are completely suppressed, so that it is often feasible to mechanically ventilate the lungs without muscle relaxations, thereby giving the anaesthetist the reassurance that if the hypnotic dose is insufficient, the patient will be able to let him know by moving (or by leaving the operating theatre in extreme circumstances!). Use of depth of anaesthesia monitors in these circumstances can also be reassuring, and may help to reduce the dose of hypnotic anaesthetic agent, reduce costs and improve cardiovascular stability.

Postoperative analgesia after remifentanil infusions

Commonly used target concentrations of remifentanil will prevent responses to all but the most severe of surgical stimuli, but within minutes of the infusion stopping the patient will revert from having profound analgesia to none at all. If an infusion of remifentanil is used with a hypnotic to maintain anaesthesia during a procedure that is likely to result in significant postoperative pain, then it is very important to ensure that adequate longer-acting measures have been taken to treat pain once the infusion of remifentanil has been switched off, otherwise the patient is likely to wake up in severe pain.

The options for ensuring analgesia on return of consciousness include one or more of the following: simple analgesics (e.g. paracetamol or non-steroidal anti-inflammatory drugs administered per rectum or via the intravenous route), wound infiltration, local or regional anaesthetic blocks, long-acting opioids such as morphine, or continuing the remifentanil infusion into the postoperative period. If morphine is to be used for postoperative analgesia then it is important to administer an intravenous bolus dose at least 40 minutes before the end of the anaesthetic. Munoz and colleagues administered standard doses of morphine at different intervals before the end of laparoscopic cholecystectomy in 120 adults, and found that pain scores and rescue analgesia requirements were significantly lower in those who received their morphine > 40 minutes before the end of surgery.[227]

In general, unless patients are to undergo a period of sedation and postoperative mechanical ventilation, postoperative remifentanil infusions are not practical and safe. The main problem is the narrow therapeutic index. Remifentanil has potent respiratory depressant effects – respiratory drive is reduced, and airway reflexes are obtunded – so that it is difficult to achieve a balance between adequate analgesia, and a patient who continues breathing. A solution to this problem is to give the patient some degree of control over the administration of the drug. While patient-controlled administration of remifentanil boluses has been successfully used in patients experiencing intermittent pain such as labour pains[228-230] the short-duration of action makes boluses unsuitable for post-surgical pain. A patient-maintained analgesia system, similar in concept to the patient-maintained sedation systems mentioned earlier, have been developed and used successfully under experimental conditions for control of pain during burns dressing changes,[231] and for control of pain after major spinal surgery,[232] cardiac surgery,[233 234] and orthopaedic surgery. As with patient-maintained sedation these systems combine patient-controlled technology with target-controlled infusion technology. When the system is activated it starts a remifentanil or alfentanil TCI at a pre-set target concentration. After that, if the patient presses an activating button the system increases the target concentration. If he does not press the button for a period of time, then the system slowly reduces the target concentration, thereby maintaining safety.

Practical precautions and pitfalls

The recently published guidelines for safe practice of TIVA contains valuable advice on the practical steps that can be taken to improve the safety of TIVA administration.[215] Some of the important principles are given here below.

DEDICATED CANNULA

When administering intravenous anaesthesia, it is advisable to administer the anaesthetic agents through a dedicated intravenous cannula. The danger of administering the drugs via a cannula that is also being used for intravenous fluids is that the rate of administration depends on the flow of the fluids, and the "dead-space" in the administration set (i.e. the internal volume of administration set distal to the point where the drugs join the intravenous fluid flow). If the intravenous fluids run out, and the dead-space volume is significant, the patient may not receive any anaesthetic agent for several minutes. A more serious problem can arise if the resistance to flow through the cannula increases, and the intravenous fluids are being administered passively (under the influence of gravity). In these situations, the drug may then flow "away from the patient" towards the intravenous fluid container, and it may take many minutes before the anaesthetist notices this. In both circumstances, there is a serious risk of awareness while drug delivery is interrupted. Once the problem is recognised, and the anaesthetist has attached a new bag of intravenous fluid or relieved an obstruction, the patient will receive a bolus of the anaesthetic drugs that were occupying the dead-space volume and the fluid administration set and if this bolus is large then adverse haemodynamic effects may result.

If it is necessary to co-administer fluids and drugs via the same cannula then it is a good idea to use a one-way valve in the fluid administration set (proximal to the point at which the drugs join the flow) to prevent the drugs from flowing the wrong way.

When a dedicated cannula or a central line is used, and it has a large bore and/or a large dead-space, then it is important to remember that at the end of the case the residual drug in the dead-space should be withdrawn, or the lines should be flushed, before the patient is returned to the post-anaesthetic care area. Failing this, if the post-anaesthesia staff are unaware of the problem and administer another drug or fluid via the same line, a significant bolus may be given with potentially serious adverse effects such as loss of consciousness and/or respiratory depression.

ADMINISTRATION SETS

Numerous varieties of intravenous anaesthetic agent administration sets are available. For situations where two or more drugs are being infused it is best to purchase sets designed for this purpose. These sets are usually constructed of a rigid material (low compliance), have low internal volume, and have anti-syphon valves close on the pump ends of the lines. Also desirable are one-way valves in the tubing from each pump to prevent reflux of one drug towards the pump for the other, and a side port to enable co-administration of another agent or even intravenous fluids should that be necessary. Ideally the lines from the different pumps should be lightly bonded to each other for the sake and tidiness and ease of use. Ready-made sets can often be purchased for less than the cost of the individual components thereby saving money and time.

SINGLE PATIENT USE

Current regulations stipulate that any ampoule or vial of anaesthetic agent is for single patient use. Intravenous anaesthetic agent disposables such as administration lines, three-way tapes and one-way valves are all strictly for single patient use.

MIXING TWO OR MORE DRUGS IN ONE SYRINGE

With the possible exception of the addition of lignocaine to propofol to reduce pain in the arm on induction of anaesthesia, there are few situations where drug mixtures can be recommended.

While there may be anecdotal reports of success with use of hypnotic and opiate mixtures there are pitfalls associated with this practise. The first is that when two drugs are mixed the mixture is legally regarded as a new, unlicensed drug, for which the anaesthetist assumes all liability. The second is that the agents may not be pharmaceutically compatible – causing one or both drugs to precipitate – or unstable. When remifentanil is added to propofol resulting in a remifentanil concentration of < 5 µg/ml in the propofol solution, the remifentanil becomes unstable and breaks down in the syringe.[236] Further, when remifentanil and propofol are mixed they undergo separation and layering, which results in variations in remifentanil concentrations across the syringe.[237] Finally, it is very unlikely that any two anaesthetic agents will have identical pharmacokinetic properties. Thus if for example a target-controlled infusion device is used, in an attempt to provide a target concentration of one component of the mixture, problems may arise when the target is increased or decreased. On an increase, the bolus dose of the second drug may be very large, whereas, when the target is decreased, and the infusion stops for a period of time, if the second drug is metabolised at a greater rate than the first, then the plasma and effect-site concentrations of the second drug may fall to excessively low levels.

METHODS TO AVOID 'SYRINGE SWAP' ERRORS

'Syringe swap' errors result in one or more pumps being programmed to administer the wrong drug. A particularly dangerous error is when propofol 1% is administered by a pump programmed to infuse remifentanil 50 µg/ml, and remifentanil 50 µg/ml is administered by a pump programmed to infuse propofol 1%. In this scenario, at standard target concentrations, a patient will be likely to receive >500 µg of remifentanil, but only 20 – 30 mg of propofol, leaving the anaesthetist with a patient who is awake, but bradycardic, hypotensive and apnoeic with a wooden chest, making bag-mask ventilation difficult.

In most operating rooms, when multiple syringe pumps are used they are mounted on a pole or other stacking system vertically one above the other. When more than one drug is to be administered by infusion, and especially when more than one drug is to be administered by TCI, then it is useful for a department to have an agreed convention stating the order of the infusion pumps. In the case of our hospital, we have agreed that the propofol pump is always on top, and that the opioid infusion pump is always second from top.

Other measures that can be taken include only programming the pumps after the labelled syringes have been loaded in the pumps (to provide the visual prompt provided by the labels and the white colour of the propofol) and double checking of the programming of the pumps (patient characteristics and model selected) before starting the infusions.

DRUG CONCENTRATIONS

In general it is good practise where possible, to always use syringes containing the same concentrations of drugs for all patients, whether administering boluses or infusions manually, or administering target-controlled infusions.

When manual administration is used, and the anaesthetist is required to calculate a bolus size or infusion rate, errors are more likely if an unfamiliar concentration is present in the syringe.

The first generation TCI pumps comprised a syringe recognition system, capable of recognising whether the pump had been loaded with a pre-filled syringe containing 1 or 2% of propofol. This made it impossible to inadvertently administer the wrong concentration of propofol by TCI (it was also impossible to administer any other drug by TCI).

The current generation of TCI pumps no longer have any facility to recognise the drug and concentration being delivered. It is therefore sensible that departments agree and only stock standard concentrations of propofol, and agree and only use standard concentrations of remifentanil and/or sufentanil for use by infusion.

CONCENTRATED DRUG SOLUTIONS, AND LOW TARGET CONCENTRATIONS AND/OR SMALL PATIENTS

Most modern infusion pumps used in the operating theatres are syringe drivers. In essence, the system recognises the diameter of the syringe, and for a given infusion rate calculates the distance that the plunger has to be pushed in per unit of time to infuse at that rate (this distance is inversely proportional to the square of the radius of the syringe). The distance the plunger should be displaced over a unit of time is then "translated" into an angular velocity or a quantity of completed rotations per unit of time of the driving motor, and the slower the angular rotation, the less accurate the rate of infusion becomes over small units of time. These and other factors limit the precision of most pumps to 0.1 mg/hr.

During target-controlled infusions the system keeps a track of the total volume infused in each period of time, by monitoring the number of rotations of the motor. At the end of each 10 second epoch the system calculates the difference between the dose that should have been administered and what was administered, and makes an allowance to correct for any error during the following epoch – this is why the infusion rate is often seen to "oscillate" between two different infusion rates while the target concentration is kept constant. The slower the infusion rate the greater the relative size of these oscillations. If a concentrated drug solution is used, then small errors in infusion rate during an epoch may result in larger (but still generally clinically insignificant) oscillating errors in the plasma concentration.

When the required infusion rate is small (as with low target concentrations or small patients), and a concentrated drug solution is used, it is wise to select the smallest syringe size practical, to maximise the displacement of the syringe plunger required. It is also important to use good quality syringes. When the infusion rate and the angular rotation of the motor are slow, the quality of the syringe becomes very important. If the rubber stopper is very compressible, or the lubricant between the stopper and the side walls of the syringe is poorly or unevenly applied, then the stopper may move in small steps rather than continuously, in effect administering a series of boluses rather than an infusion. Use of a good quality small syringe will thus improve the accuracy and stability of the infusion rate.

5
—
The future

In recent years, competition from generic versions of propofol and some of the older opioid analgesics, has caused significant reductions in the costs of these drugs. New and more robust pharmacokinetic-dynamics models have been published. Various medical device companies have launched (or will launch in the near future) new products and new medical device companies have entered into the TCI business.

As more anaesthetists gain access to TCI systems for these agents, and environmental concerns mount, it is likely that the popularity and frequency of use of intravenous anaesthesia in general, and target-controlled infusions in particular, will increase. Now that TIVA has become established in adult practice it is likely they it will increasingly be used in children, who will also be able to enjoy the benefits of TIVA and TCI.

NEW, IMPROVED MODELS

Most models in use at present work best for healthy adults, but do not apply to, or perform poorly when used for young, elderly or unwell patients. Although more sophisticated models for use in special populations (young, elderly) have been published, few studies have validated the predictive performance of TCI systems in these groups. This is likely to change with time. We might see models that apply to these specific groups, or general models that can take into account more of the co-variates such as age, that are responsible for the inter-patient pharmacokinetic variability. New models, or improvements to current models are likely to be associated with more accurate control of targeted plasma and effect-site drug concentrations.

The current trend of an increasing incidence of obesity is likely to be maintained. As older body size descriptors such as lean body mass (applied in the Schnider and Minto model) doesn't cope with the population at the extremes, better solutions have been studied. An example is the allometric scaling based on predicted fat-free mass (FFM) implemented in the new models for propofol, remifentanil and dexmedetomidine. The interested reader is referred to the on-line supplement entitled "explorations of scaling functions"[2] which accompanies the publication by Eleveld et al. and which describes the development of the general purpose remifentanil model.[64] Further research into the pharmacokinetics of anaesthetic drugs in the obese is required, as are studies specifically investigating the performance of the current models in the obese.

NEW DRUGS

No new volatile anaesthetic agents have been discovered within the last few decades. In the future, it is likely that there will be pressure from governments and regulatory authorities to reduce the usage of agents with harmful environmental effects, and this might cause a decline in the use of volatile anaesthetic agents, which would in turn stimulate the development and use of newer, safe intravenous agents.

None of the currently available intravenous anaesthetic agents are perfect. Hopefully new, drugs such as ABP-700[238 239] and remimazolam[240] with improved pharmacokinetic and pharmacodynamic profiles will be introduced in the market for anesthesia and sedation.[241] Ideally, one day we will have short-acting agents that cause anxiolysis without sedation and respiratory depression, analgesics that don't cause nausea and vomiting and hypnotics that don't cause pain on injection and cardio-respiratory compromise.

PATIENT-CONTROLLED TCI SYSTEMS

Patient-controlled TCI systems, when used for sedation and analgesia, have been popular[242] with patients, surgeons and anaesthetists, and bring potential improvements in safety and patient satisfaction. It is likely that patient-control functionality will be added to commercially available TCI pumps in the not-too-distant future.

TARGET-CONTROLLED INFUSION FOR OTHER DRUGS

The knowledge obtained from TCI applications in anaesthesia could be extrapolated to other areas of medicine. Recently, Colin et al. investigated the clinical utility of target-controlled infusions of antibiotics in an intensive care unit setting using vancomycin as a model compound.[243] They compared target-controlled

---

2 https://download.lww.com/wolterskluwer_vitalstream_com/PermaLink/ALN/B/
ALN_2017_03_15_ELEVELD_ALN-D-15-01316_SDC1.pdf (accessed 7 July 2019)

infusion and adaptive target-controlled infusion, which combines target-controlled infusion with data from therapeutic drug monitoring, with conventional (therapeutic drug monitoring-based) vancomycin dosing strategies and concluded that adaptive target-controlled infusion has the potential to become a practical tool for patient-tailored antibiotic dosing in the intensive care unit.

ADVISORY DISPLAYS GUIDING TCI TARGETS

Integrating all sources of pharmacologic information including that from past drug interaction studies, along with real time measurements of the patient responses to a specific drug dose might offer a powerful advisory tool to depict the complete dose-response relationship of multiple drugs, thereby optimizing drug administration and improving patient care. Systems such as Smart Pilot View (Dräger, Lübeck, Germany), GE Navigator Applications Suite (GE Healthcare, Chicago, Il, USA) and Medvis Anesthesia Diplays (Medvis, Salt Lake City, Utah, USA) are such systems displaying the effect-site concentrations of combined drugs (opioids and intravenous or inhalation hypnotics), based on pharmacokinetic models and the resulting anaesthetic effect and on pharmacodynamic models. Effects are depicted as population-based probabilities of unconsciousness, absent responses to tracheal intubation, and other clinical pharmacodynamic endpoints.[167]

CLOSED LOOP CONTROL OF ANAESTHESIA

Various processed EEG variables such as the Bispectral Index have been used by computerised systems to automatically control TCI infusions of propofol for sedation and general anaesthesia.[244-246] These systems have the potential to provide more accurate control of anaesthesia. For optimal function closed-loop systems require control variables that accurately reflect the process being controlled. Progress with our understanding of the process of anaesthesia, coupled with improved measures of anaesthetic depth could see increased use of computer control of anaesthesia.

ONLINE PROPOFOL MEASUREMENTS

Recently, a point of care propofol analyser has been developed that can provide accurate plasma propofol measurements within 4 minutes.[17 247] Different research groups are currently developing online methods of assaying exhaled concentrations of propofol metabolites,[12-14 248 249] from which it is possible to estimate plasma propofol concentrations.[15 16 250] There is already a commercially available monitor that provides one estimate of plasma propofol concentration per minute.

Such rapidly acquired measurements can be used to identify patients in whom the individual pharmacokinetics do not conform well with a population model being used for TCI propofol administration,[251] and this information might for example explain unexpected haemodynamic instability and inform further clinical decision making. A further logical step is to use this information to adapt the model in use during the infusion.[252]

6
—
Case studies

Case 1: Moderate to deep sedation for gastroscopic resection of oesophageal lesions (adenocarcinoma)

History:
The patient was a 70 year old male (173 cm, 89 kg, ASA status 2), who suffered from an oesophageal carcinoma. His medical history consisted of hypertension, well controlled with beta-blockers, and diabetis mellitus type II treated with metformin.

Surgical procedure:
Gastroscopic resection of oesophageal lesions (adenocarcinoma).

Sedation management:
While routine physiological monitoring was commenced (3 lead ECG, non-invasive blood pressure, SaO_2, end-tidal CO_2 and respiration rate), an intravenous cannula was inserted and a crystalloid infusion commenced. Paracetamol 1000 mg iv was given just after induction. Supplementary oxygen (2 l/min) was given by nasal cannulae. An effect-compartment targeted TCI of remifentanil (Minto model) was commenced at a target of 1 ng/ml. Two minutes later, propofol effect-compartment TCI (Schnider model with fixed tpeak) commenced with an initial target of 2 µg/ml. At intervals of 90 seconds (consistent with the time to peak effect of 1.6 minutes), the propofol target concentration was increased to 2.3 µg/ml and then to 2.6 µg/ml whereupon a level of moderate to deep sedation appropriate for this procedure was reached. Five minutes after the start of infusions, the gastroscope was successfully inserted and the endoscopic procedure commenced. Later an excessive level of analgosedation occurred, inducing decreases in blood pressure and respiratory rate, and airway obstruction requiring a chin-lift manoeuvre. The propofol target was decreased to 2.2 µg/ml at 18 min-

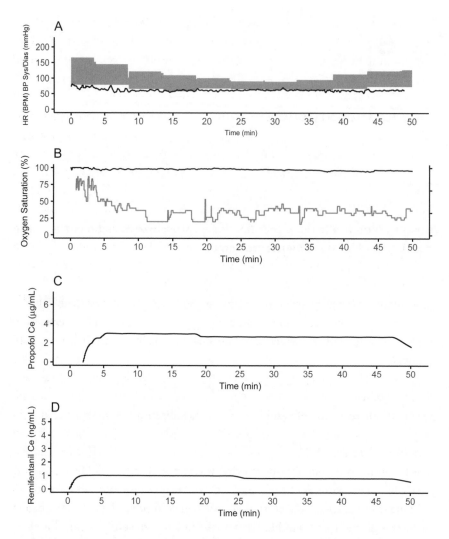

Figure 11: Anaesthesia record for moderate to deep sedation during a gastroscopic resection of oesophageal lesions. Panel A: heart rate (black line) and non-invasive blood pressure (grey zone); Panel B: SpO2 (black line), Respiratory rate (grey line); Panel C: Propofol effect-site concentrations (Schnider model with fixed tpeak); Panel D: Remifentanil effect-site concentrations (Minto model).

utes and the remifentanil target was decreased to 0.8 ng/ml at 23 minutes. Both drug infusions were stopped at the end of the case (after 48 minutes). The patient breathed spontaneously throughout the procedure and woke up 5 minutes after the drug infusions were stopped. Recovery was uneventful and he returned home the same day.

Case 2: Anaesthesia for a resection of a malignant fibromyxoid sarcoma of the elbow combined with an intra-operative, isolated single limb perfusion with cytostatics

History:

The patient was a 55 year old male (181 cm, 105 kg, ASA II), who suffered from a calcifying fibromyxoid sarcoma arising from the elbow requiring resection and intra-operative, isolated single limb perfusion with cytostatics (TNF and melphalan). His medical history consists of some elevated blood pressure still not considered hypertension (no medication required).

Procedure:

While routine physiological monitoring was commenced (5 lead ECG, heart rate, non-invasive blood pressure, SaO_2, capnography, depth of anaesthesia monitoring measured by qCON and BIS, responsiveness monitoring measured by qNOX) an intravenous cannula was inserted and a crystalloid infusion was commenced (8 ml/kg/h). Antibiotics (cephazoline 2000 mg) were administered prior to induction of anaesthesia. After preoxygenation for 5 minutes, anaesthesia was induced with an effect-site targeted TCI of remifentanil (Minto model) at an initial target of 4 ng/ml. Two minutes later, effect-site targeted TCI of propofol (Schnider model with fixed tpeak) was started at an initial target of 2 μg/ml in order to avoid to a rapid fall in blood pressure. As shown in Panel B of the figure, this propofol concentration had only a small effect on the BIS and qCON values indicating a marginal cerebral drug effect. Therefore, propofol targets were increased stepwise to 5 and 6 after 90 and 180 seconds, respectively, hereby taking into account the time required to reach pseudo-steady state after every increase. A bolus of rocuronium (0.60 mg/kg) followed by a continuous infusion of rocuronium (0.3 mg/kg/h) was given. Five minutes after the start of the propofol infusion, the trachea was intubated and pressure-controlled ventilation was started. An arterial line was inserted in the right radial artery and a central venous catheter was inserted in the right internal jugular vein. Thereafter, the propofol and remifentanil concentrations could be decreased and were targeted to maintain depth of anaesthesia measures (BIS and qCON) between 40 and 50 and haemodynamic parameters and the responsiveness index (qNOX) within clinical range. After the resection of the tumor and before cannulation of the brachial artery and vein, a bolus of heparin 5000 IE was administered. Additional crystalloid fluids and a continuous infusion of noradrenaline were administered in order to maintain a high enough blood pressure (at least 20 mmHg above perfusion pressure of the single-limb perfusion) to avoid

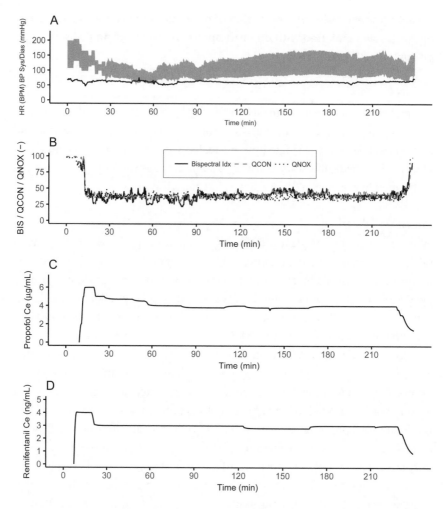

Figure 12: Anaesthesia record for resection of a malignant calcifying fibromyxoid sarcoma of the elbow combined with an intra-operative, isolated single limb perfusion with cytostatics. Panel A: heart rate (black line) and non-invasive/invasive blood pressure (grey zone); Panel B: depth of anaesthesia indices BIS (bispectral index, Medtronic, USA) and qCON (CONOX monitor, Fresenius, France) and qNOX responsiveness index (CONOX monitor, Fresenius, France); Panel C: Propofol effect-site concentrations (Schnider model with fixed tpeak); Panel D: Remifentanil effect-site concentrations (Minto model).

leakage of the cytostatics from the isolated limb into the systemic circulation. The rocuronium infusion was stopped 30 minutes before the end of surgery (after termination of single-limb perfusion), and protamine 10000 IE administered after removal of the cannula. Paracetamol 1000 mg and diclofenac 75 mg, morphine 0.07 mg/kg morphine and ondansetron 4 mg was given 30 minutes prior to the end of surgery (at starting skin closure). At skin closure, a bolus sugammadex 2 mg/kg was administered to avoid residual muscle paralysis. Infusions of propofol and remifentanil were stopped at skin closure. The noradrenaline infusion was gradually decreased after the termination of the perfusion and stopped just before recovery. The patient woke up within the next few minutes and was transferred to the PACU. Recovery was uneventful and he was transferred to the ward the next day, and discharged home a few days later.

Case 3: Anaesthesia for a laparotomy (rectovaginoplasty)

History:

The patient was an 83 year old female patient (154 cm, 52 kg, ASA 3) with a medical history of diabetis mellitus (insulin dependent), early stage dementia, hypertension and heart failure (well controlled with amlodipine and irbesartan), hypercholesterolemia (atorvastatin), and vertigo (betahistine). She used benzodiazepines daily (temazepam 10 mg). She suffered from extensive pelvic organ prolapse requiring rectovaginoplasty through a laparotomy.

Procedure:

Routine physiological monitoring was commenced (5 lead ECG, heart rate, non-invasive blood pressure, SaO_2, capnography, BIS) and an intravenous cannula was inserted and a crystalloid infusion was commenced (4-6 ml/kg/h). An epidural catheter (L2-L3) was inserted and epidural analgesia was started with a 10ml bolus of ropivacaine 0.375%, and a continuous infusion of ropivacaine 2mg/ml and sufentanil 1μg/ml (infusion rate 6 ml/h). Cephazoline 2000 mg was administered prior to induction of anaesthesia. After preoxygenation for 5 minutes, anaesthesia was induced with effect-site targeted TCI of sufentanil (Gepts model) at an initial target of 0.25 ng/ml. Four minutes later, effect-site targeted TCI of propofol (Eleveld PKPD model) was started at an initial target of 2.27 μg/ml, being the patient-individualized predicted EC50 (concentration required for a BIS of 47). As shown in Panel B, the patient lost consciousness and reached an accurate BIS with these target concentrations. Rocuronium iv 0.6 mg/kg was given after loss of consciousness and the patient's trachea was intubated and pressure-controlled ventilation was started. An arterial line was inserted in the right radial artery and a central venous catheter inserted in the right internal jugular vein. As shown in the figure, haemodynamic parameters were very stable and depth of anaesthesia was maintained with BIS values between 45 and 60 without any required change in the propofol target concentration. Two supplementary boli of rocuronium were administered, being 20 and 10 mg at minute 30 and 60, respectively. At minute 70, the sufentanil target concentration was increased to 0.3 ng/ml for a short time due to exploration of the upper abdomen (not blocked by the epidural analgesia). The sufentanil target concentration was lowered to 0.2 ng/ml at 90 minutes and to zero at 160 minutes (45 minutes before the expected end of surgery). Paracetamol 1000 mg, metamizole 1000 mg and ondansetron 4 mg were given iv. 30 minutes prior to the expected end of surgery. The propofol administration was stopped at the end of surgery and (as seen in Panel B) a very timely return of consciousness was observed. The patient

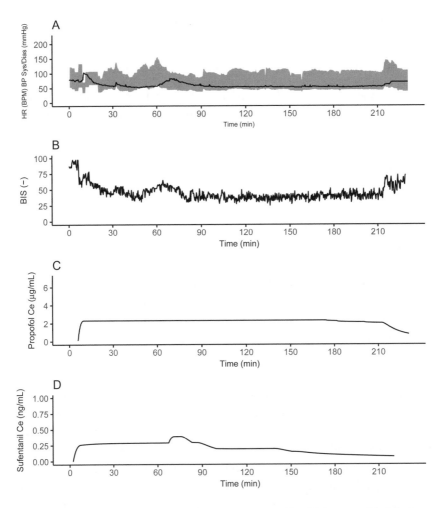

Figure 13: Anaesthesia record for laparotomy (rectovaginoplasty) Panel A: heart rate (black line) and non-invasive/invasive blood pressure (grey zone); Panel B: depth of anaesthesia indices BIS (bispectral index, Medtronic, USA); Panel C: Propofol effect-site concentrations (Eleveld PKPD model); Panel D: Remifentanil effect-site concentrations (Minto model).

was transferred to the PACU where her recovery was uneventful with low pain scores (VAS between 3 and 1). She was transferred to the ward 4 hours postoperatively and discharged home within the next days.

Case 4: Laparotomy for partial bowel resection and reconstruction of ureter

History:

The patient was a 42 year old woman with a history of severe endometriosis resulting in multiple adhesions of the intestinal structures. Recently, she had developed a colo-vesical fistula.

Surgical procedure:

Laparotomy

Anaesthetic management:

While routine physiological monitoring was commenced (5 lead ECG, heart rate, non-invasive blood pressure, SaO_2, capnography) and recorded at 5-minute intervals, an intravenous cannula was inserted and BIS electrodes (Medtronic, USA) were applied to the forehead. The electrodes were connected to a VISTA BIS monitor (Medtronic, USA). After pre-oxygenation, sufentanil effect-site targeted TCI using the Gepts model was commenced at a target concentration of 0.3 ng/ml. Two minutes later, anaesthesia was induced with a slow bolus of propofol 1 % (1.5 mg/kg). After loss of consciousness, a bolus of rocuronium 0.6 mg/kg was given to facilitate tracheal intubation. After intubation, sevoflurane was started and titrated to maintain a BIS between 40 and 50. The patients' lungs were ventilated using IPPV to maintain normocapnia. A heating system was used to maintain normothermia, and a urinary catheter was inserted to monitor urine output. The sufentanil target concentration was titrated to maintain stable haemodynamic parameters. A central venous line was inserted in the internal jugular vein to administer fluids and measure central venous pressure (CVP). Prophylactic antibiotics were given. During the case, intermittent bolus doses of rocuronium were given when required. Details are plotted in the figure.

Forty-five minutes before the predicted end of surgery the sufentanil infusion was stopped. Intravenous paracetamol (1g) and morphine 0.15 mg/kg were given to provide postoperative pain relief. During skin closure (when the effect-site sufentanil concentration was 0.1 ng/ml) the patient started breathing spontaneously. After skin closure, sevoflurane administration was stopped and the endotracheal tube was removed after return of consciousness. The patient was transferred to the postoperative recovery room, where a morphine intravenous PCA system was connected. The patient remained in the PACU for 24 hours and returned to the ward for further recovery. The postoperative phase was uneventful.

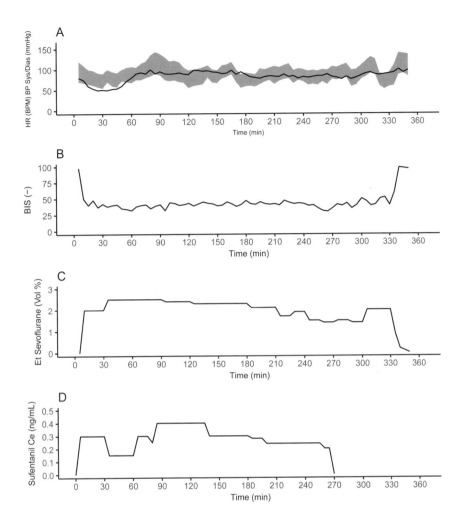

Figure 14: Anaesthesia record for laparotomy for partial bowel resection and reconstruction of ureter. Panel A: heart rate (black line) and non-invasive/invasive blood pressure measured every 5 minutes (grey zone); Panel B: depth of anaesthesia indices BIS (bispectral index, Medtronic, USA); Panel C: end-tidal sevoflurane concentration (Zeus ventilator Dräger, Germany in autoflow modus using end-tidal targeted inhaled drug administration); Panel D: Sufentanil target effect-site concentrations (Gepts model).

References

1   Doze VA, Westphal LM, White PF. Comparison of propofol with methohexital for outpatient anesthesia. *Anesth Analg* 1986;65:1189-95.

2   Lim BL, Low TC. Total intravenous anaesthesia versus inhalational anaesthesia for dental day surgery. *Anaesth Intensive Care* 1992;20(4):475-8.

3   Borgeat A, Wilder Smith OH, Saiah M, et al. Subhypnotic doses of propofol relieve pruritus induced by epidural and intrathecal morphine. *Anesthesiology* 1992;76:510-12.

4   Eriksson H, Korttila K. Recovery profile after desflurane with or without ondansetron compared with propofol in patients undergoing outpatient gynecological laparoscopy. *Anesth Analg* 1996;82(3):533-38.

5   Hartung J. Twenty-four of twenty-seven studies show a greater incidence of emesis associated with nitrous oxide than with alternative anesthetics. *Anesth Analg* 1996;83(1):114-16.

6   Raeder J, Gupta A, Pedersen FM. Recovery characteristics of sevoflurane- or propofol-based anaesthesia for day-care surgery. *Acta Anaesthesiol Scand* 1997;41(8):988-94.

7   James MF. Nitrous oxide: still useful in the year 2000? *Curr Opin Anaesthesiol* 1999;12(4):461-66.

8   Sukhani R, Lurie J, Jabamoni R. Propofol for ambulatory gynecologic laparoscopy: does omission of nitrous oxide alter postoperative emetic sequelae and recovery? *Anesth Analg* 1994;78(5):831-35.

9   Smith I, Terhoeve PA, Hennart D, et al. A multicentre comparison of the costs of anaesthesia with sevoflurane or propofol. *Br J Anaesth* 1999;83(4):564-70.

10 Sherman J, Le C, Lamers V, et al. Life cycle greenhouse gas emissions of anesthetic drugs. *Anesth Analg* 2012;114(5):1086-90.

11 Stockholm county council. Environmentally classified pharmaceuticals [Available from: http://www.janusinfo.se/environment accessed 21 April, 2019.

12 Perl T, Carstens E, Hirn A, et al. Determination of serum propofol concentrations by breath analysis using ion mobility spectrometry. *Br J Anaesth* 2009;103(6):822-27.

13 Grossherr M, Hengstenberg A, Meier T, et al. Propofol concentration in exhaled air and arterial plasma in mechanically ventilated patients undergoing cardiac surgery. *Br J Anaesth* 2009;102(5):608-13.

14 Hornuss C, Wiepcke D, Praun S, et al. Time course of expiratory propofol after bolus injection as measured by ion molecule reaction mass spectrometry. *Analytical and bioanalytical chemistry* 2012;403(2):555-61.

15 Kreuer S, Hauschild A, Fink T, et al. Two different approaches for pharmacokinetic modeling of exhaled drug concentrations. *Sci Rep* 2014;4:5423.

16 Colin P, Eleveld DJ, van den Berg JP, et al. Propofol Breath Monitoring as a Potential Tool to Improve the Prediction of Intraoperative Plasma Concentrations. *Clin Pharmacokinet* 2016;55(7):849-59.

17 Cowley NJ, Laitenberger P, Liu B, et al. Evaluation of a new analyser for rapid measurement of blood propofol concentration during cardiac surgery. *Anaesthesia* 2012;67(8):870-74.

18 Struys MM, De Smet T, Glen JI, et al. The History of Target-Controlled Infusion. *Anesth Analg* 2016;122(1):56-69.

19 Kruger-Thiemer E. Continuous intravenous infusion and multicompartment accumulation. *Eur J Pharmacol* 1968;4(3):317-24.

20 Vaughan DP, Tucker GT. General theory for rapidly establishing steady state drug concentrations using two consecutive constant rate intravenous infusions. *Eur J Clin Pharmacol* 1975;9(2-3):235-38.

21 Vaughan DP, Tucker GT. General derivation of the ideal intravenous drug input required to achieve and maintain a constant plasma drug concentration. Theoretical application to lignocaine therapy. *Eur J Clin Pharmacol* 1976;10(6):433-40.

22 Schwilden H. A general method for calculating the dosage scheme in linear pharmacokinetics. *Eur J Clin Pharmacol* 1981;20(5):379-86.

23 Alvis JM, Reves JG, Govier AV, et al. Computer-assisted continuous infusions of fentanyl during cardiac anesthesia: comparison with a manual method. *Anesthesiology* 1985;63(1):41-49.

24 Crankshaw DP, Boyd MD, Bjorksten AR. Plasma drug efflux--a new approach to optimization of drug infusion for constant blood concentration of thiopental and methohexital. *Anesthesiology* 1987;67(1):32-41.

25 Tavernier A, Coussaert E, d'Hollander A, et al. Model-based pharmacokinetic regulation in computer-assisted anesthesia an interactive system: CARIN. *Acta Anaesthesiol Belg* 1987;38(1):63-8.

26 Shafer SL, Siegel LC, Cooke JE, et al. Testing computer-controlled infusion pumps by simulation. *Anesthesiology* 1988;68(2):261-6.

27 Jacobs JR. Algorithm for optimal linear model-based control with application to pharmacokinetic model-driven drug delivery. *IEEE Trans Biomed Eng* 1990;37(1):107-9.

28 Shafer SL, Gregg KM. Algorithms to rapidly achieve and maintain stable drug concentrations at the site of drug effect with a computer-controlled infusion pump. *J Pharmacokinet Biopharm* 1992;20(2):147-69.

29 Jacobs JR, Williams EA. Algorithm to control effect compartment drug concentrations in pharmacokinetic model-driven drug delivery. *IEEE Trans Biomed Eng* 1993;40(10):993-9.

30 Absalom AR, Glen JB, Zwart GJC, et al. Target-Controlled Infusion: A Mature Technology. *Anesth Analg* 2016;122(1):70-78.

31 Ausems ME, Stanski DR, Hug CC. An evaluation of the accuracy of pharmacokinetic data for the computer assisted infusion of alfentanil. *Br J Anaesth* 1985;57(12):1217-25.

32 Glass PS, Jacobs JR, Smith LR, et al. Pharmacokinetic model-driven infusion of fentanyl: assessment of accuracy. *Anesthesiology* 1990;73(6):1082-90.

33 Shafer SL, Varvel JR, Aziz N, et al. Pharmacokinetics of fentanyl administered by computer-controlled infusion pump. *Anesthesiology* 1990;73(6):1091-102.

34 Chaudhri S, White M, Kenny GN. Induction of anaesthesia with propofol using a target-controlled infusion system. *Anaesthesia* 1992;47(7):551-53.

35 Glass PS, Glen JB, Kenny GN, et al. Nomenclature for computer-assisted infusion devices. *Anesthesiology* 1997;86(6):1430-1.

36 Glen JB. The development of 'Diprifusor': a TCI system for propofol. *Anaesthesia* 1998;53 Suppl 1:13-21.

37 Gray JM, Kenny GN. Development of the technology for 'Diprifusor' TCI systems. *Anaesthesia* 1998;53 Suppl 1:22-7.

38 Taylor I, White M, Kenny GN. Assessment of the value and pattern of use of a target controlled propofol infusion system. *Int J Clin Monit Comput* 1993;10(3):175-80.

39 Russell D, Wilkes MP, Hunter SC, et al. Manual compared with target-controlled infusion of propofol. *Br J Anaesth* 1995;75(5):562-66.

40 Servin FS. TCI compared with manually controlled infusion of propofol: a multicentre study. *Anaesthesia* 1998;53 Suppl 1:82-86.

41 Glen JB. Quality of anaesthesia during spontaneous respiration: a proposed scoring system. *Anaesthesia* 1991;46(12):1081-2.

42 Struys M, Versichelen L, Rolly G. Influence of pre-anaesthetic medication on target propofol concentration using a 'Diprifusor' TCI system during ambulatory surgery. *Anaesthesia* 1998;53 Suppl 1:68-71:68-71.

43 Barvais L, Rausin I, Glen JB, et al. Administration of propofol by target-controlled infusion in patients undergoing coronary artery surgery. *J Cardiothorac Vasc Anesth* 1996;10(7):877-83.

44 Swinhoe CF, Peacock JE, Glen JB, et al. Evaluation of the predictive performance of a 'Diprifusor' TCI system. *Anaesthesia* 1998;53 Suppl 1:61-7.

45 Richards AL, Orton JK, Gregory MJ. Influence of ventilatory mode on target concentrations required for anaesthesia using a 'Diprifusor' TCI system. *Anaesthesia* 1998;53 Suppl 1:77-81.

46 Servin FS, Marchand-Maillet F, Desmonts JM. Influence of analgesic supplementation on the target propofol concentrations for anaesthesia with 'Diprifusor' TCI. *Anaesthesia* 1998;53 Suppl 1:72-76.

47 Mu J, Jiang T, Xu XB, et al. Comparison of target-controlled infusion and manual infusion for propofol anaesthesia in children. *Br J Anaesth* 2018;120(5):1049-55.

48 Leslie K, Clavisi O, Hargrove J. Target-controlled infusion versus manually-controlled infusion of propofol for general anaesthesia or sedation in adults. *Cochrane Database Syst Rev* 2008(3):CD006059.

49 Shafer SL, Varvel JR, Gronert GA. A comparison of parametric with semiparametric analysis of the concentration versus effect relationship of metocurine in dogs and pigs. *J Pharmacokinet Biopharm* 1989;17(3):291-304.

50 Coppens MJ, Eleveld DJ, Proost JH, et al. An evaluation of using population pharmacokinetic models to estimate pharmacodynamic parameters for propofol and bispectral index in children. *Anesthesiology* 2011;115(1):83-93.

51 Mertens MJ, Engbers FH, Burm AG, et al. Predictive performance of computer-controlled infusion of remifentanil during propofol/remifentanil anaesthesia. *British Journal of Anaesthesia* 2003;90(2):132-41.

52 Marsh B, White M, Morton N, et al. Pharmacokinetic model driven infusion of propofol in children. *Br J Anaesth* 1991;67:41-48.

53 Schnider TW, Minto CF, Gambus PL, et al. The influence of method of administration and covariates on the pharmacokinetics of propofol in adult volunteers. *Anesthesiology* 1998;88(5):1170-82.

54 Schnider TW, Minto CF, Shafer SL, et al. The influence of age on propofol pharmacodynamics. *Anesthesiology* 1999;90(6):1502-16.

55 Minto CF, Schnider TW, Egan TD, et al. Influence of age and gender on the pharmacokinetics and pharmacodynamics of remifentanil. I. Model development. *Anesthesiology* 1997;86(1):10-23.

56 Minto CF, Schnider TW, Shafer SL. Pharmacokinetics and pharmacodynamics of remifentanil. II. Model application. *Anesthesiology* 1997;86(1):24-33.

57 Eleveld DJ, Colin P, Absalom AR, et al. Pharmacokinetic-pharmacodynamic model for propofol for broad application in anaesthesia and sedation. *Br J Anaesth* 2018;120(5):942-59.

58 Minto CF, Schnider TW, Gregg KM, et al. Using the time of maximum effect site concentration to combine pharmacokinetics and pharmacodynamics. *Anesthesiology* 2003;99(2):324-33.

59 Hannivoort LN, Eleveld DJ, Proost JH, et al. Development of an Optimized Pharmacokinetic Model of Dexmedetomidine Using Target-Controlled Infusion in Healthy Volunteers. *Anesthesiology* 2015;123(2):357-67.

60 Eleveld DJ, Proost JH, Absalom AR, et al. Obesity and allometric scaling of pharmacokinetics. *Clin Pharmacokinet* 2011;50(11):751-3.

61 Kataria BK, Ved SA, Nicodemus HF, et al. The pharmacokinetics of propofol in children using three different data analysis approaches. *Anesthesiology* 1994;80(1):104-22.

62 Absalom A, Amutike D, Lal A, et al. Accuracy of the 'Paedfusor' in children undergoing cardiac surgery or catheterization. *Br J Anaesth* 2003;91(4):507-13.

63 Absalom A, Kenny G. 'Paedfusor' pharmacokinetic data set. *Br J Anaesth* 2005;95(1):110.

64 Eleveld DJ, Proost JH, Vereecke H, et al. An Allometric Model of Remifentanil Pharmacokinetics and Pharmacodynamics. *Anesthesiology* 2017;126(6):1005-18.

65 Sahinovic MM, Struys M, Absalom AR. Clinical Pharmacokinetics and Pharmacodynamics of Propofol. *Clin Pharmacokinet* 2018;57(12):1539-58.

66 Gepts E, Jonckheer K, Maes V, et al. Disposition kinetics of propofol during alfentanil anaesthesia. *Anaesthesia* 1988;43(Suppl):8-13.

67 White M, Kenny GN, Schraag S. Use of target controlled infusion to derive age and gender covariates for propofol clearance. *Clin Pharmacokinet* 2008;47(2):119-27.

68 Schuttler J, Ihmsen H. Population pharmacokinetics of propofol: a multicenter study. *Anesthesiology* 2000;92(3):727-38.

69 James W. Research on obesity. London: Her Majesty's Stationary Office, 1976.

70 Absalom AR, Mani V, De Smet T, et al. Pharmacokinetic models for propofol-defining and illuminating the devil in the detail. *Br J Anaesth* 2009;103(1):26-37.

71 Servin F, Farinotti R, Haberer JP, et al. Propofol infusion for maintenance of anesthesia in morbidly obese patients receiving nitrous oxide. A clinical and pharmacokinetic study. *Anesthesiology* 1993;78(4):657-65.

72 Wietasch JK, Scholz M, Zinserling J, et al. The performance of a target-controlled infusion of propofol in combination with remifentanil: a clinical investigation with two propofol formulations. *Anesth Analg* 2006;102(2):430-37.

73 Coetzee JF, Glen JB, Wium CA, et al. Pharmacokinetic model selection for target controlled infusions of propofol. Assessment of three parameter sets. *Anesthesiology* 1995;82(6):1328-45.

74 van Kralingen S, Diepstraten J, Peeters MY, et al. Population pharmacokinetics and pharmacodynamics of propofol in morbidly obese patients. *Clin Pharmacokinet* 2011;50(11):739-50.

75 Cortinez LI, Anderson BJ, Penna A, et al. Influence of obesity on propofol pharmacokinetics: derivation of a pharmacokinetic model. *Br J Anaesth* 2010;105(4):448-56.

76 Murat I, Billard V, Vernois J, et al. Pharmacokinetics of propofol after a single dose in children aged 1-3 years with minor burns. Comparison of three data analysis approaches. *Anesthesiology* 1996;84(3):526-32.

77 Saint-Maurice C, Cockshott ID, Douglas EJ, et al. Pharmacokinetics of propofol in young children after a single dose. *BrJAnaesth* 1989;63(6):667-70.

78 Hara M, Masui K, Eleveld DJ, et al. Predictive performance of eleven pharmacokinetic models for propofol infusion in children for long-duration anaesthesia. *Br J Anaesth* 2017;118(3):415-23.

79 Eleveld DJ, Proost JH, Cortinez LI, et al. A general purpose pharmacokinetic model for propofol. *Anesth Analg* 2014;118(6):1221-37.

80 Dershwitz M, Hoke JF, Rosow CE, et al. Pharmacokinetics and pharmacodynamics of remifentanil in volunteer subjects with severe liver disease. *Anesthesiology* 1996;84(4):812-20.

81 Hoke JF, Shlugman D, Dershwitz M, et al. Pharmacokinetics and pharmacodynamics of remifentanil in persons with renal failure compared with healthy volunteers. *Anesthesiology* 1997;87(3):533-41.

82 Rigby-Jones AE, Priston MJ, Sneyd JR, et al. Remifentanil-midazolam sedation for paediatric patients receiving mechanical ventilation after cardiac surgery. *Br J Anaesth* 2007;99(2):252-61.

83 Ross AK, Davis PJ, Dear Gd GL, et al. Pharmacokinetics of remifentanil in anesthetized pediatric patients undergoing elective surgery or diagnostic procedures. *Anesth Analg* 2001;93(6):1393-401.

84 La Colla L, Albertin A, La Colla G, et al. Predictive performance of the 'Minto' remifentanil pharmacokinetic parameter set in morbidly obese patients ensuing from a new method for calculating lean body mass. *Clin Pharmacokinet* 2010;49(2):131-39.

85 Janmahasatian S, Duffull SB, Ash S, et al. Quantification of lean bodyweight. *Clin Pharmacokinet* 2005;44(10):1051-65.

86 Kim TK, Obara S, Egan TD, et al. Disposition of Remifentanil in Obesity: A New Pharmacokinetic Model Incorporating the Influence of Body Mass. *Anesthesiology* 2017;126(6):1019-32.

87 La Colla L, Albertin A, La Colla G. Pharmacokinetic model-driven remifentanil administration in the morbidly obese: the 'critical weight' and the 'fictitious height', a possible solution to an unsolved problem? *Clin Pharmacokinet* 2009;48(6):397-98.

88 Egan TD, Huizinga B, Gupta SK, et al. Remifentanil pharmacokinetics in obese versus lean patients. *Anesthesiology* 1998;89(3):562-73.

89 Mertens MJ, Olofsen E, Engbers FH, et al. Propofol reduces perioperative remifentanil requirements in a synergistic manner: response surface modeling of perioperative remifentanil-propofol interactions. *Anesthesiology* 2003;99(2):347-59.

90 Hughes MA, Glass PS, Jacobs JR. Context-sensitive half-time in multicompartment pharmacokinetic models for intravenous anesthetic drugs. *Anesthesiology* 1992;76:334-41.

91 Gepts E, Shafer SL, Camu F, et al. Linearity of pharmacokinetics and model estimation of sufentanil. *Anesthesiology* 1995;83(6):1194-204.

92 Camu F, Gepts E, Rucquoi M, et al. Pharmacokinetics of alfentanil in man. *Anesth Analg* 1982;61(8):657-61.

93 Bower S, Hull CJ. Comparative pharmacokinetics of fentanyl and alfentanil. *Br J Anaesth* 1982;54(8):871-77.

94 Chauvin M, Bonnet F, Montembault C, et al. The influence of hepatic plasma flow on alfentanil plasma concentration plateaus achieved with an infusion model in humans: measurement of alfentanil hepatic extraction coefficient. *Anesth Analg* 1986;65(10):999-1003.

95 Bovill JG, Sebel PS, Blackburn CL, et al. The pharmacokinetics of alfentanil (R39209): a new opioid analgesic. *Anesthesiology* 1982;57(6):439-43.

96 Helmers H, Van Peer A, Woestenborghs R, et al. Alfentanil kinetics in the elderly. *Clin Pharmacol Ther* 1984;36(2):239-43.

97 Maitre PO, Vozeh S, Heykants J, et al. Population pharmacokinetics of alfentanil: the average dose-plasma concentration relationship and interindividual variability in patients. *Anesthesiology* 1987;66:3-12.

98 Hudson RJ, Thomson IR, Cannon JE, et al. Pharmacokinetics of fentanyl in patients undergoing abdominal aortic surgery. *Anesthesiology* 1986;64(3):334-38.

99 McClain DA, Hug CC, Jr. Intravenous fentanyl kinetics. *Clin Pharmacol Ther* 1980;28(1):106-14.

100 Scott JC, Stanski DR. Decreased fentanyl and alfentanil dose requirements with age. A simultaneous pharmacokinetic and pharmacodynamic evaluation. *J Pharmacol Exp Ther* 1987;240:159-66.

101 Shibutani K, Inchiosa MA, Jr., Sawada K, et al. Accuracy of pharmacokinetic models for predicting plasma fentanyl concentrations in lean and obese surgical patients: derivation of dosing weight ("pharmacokinetic mass"). *Anesthesiology* 2004;101(3):603-13.

102 Roerig DL, Kotrly KJ, Vucins EJ, et al. First pass uptake of fentanyl, meperidine, and morphine in the human lung. *Anesthesiology* 1987;67(4):466-72.

103 Weerink MAS, Struys M, Hannivoort LN, et al. Clinical Pharmacokinetics and Pharmacodynamics of Dexmedetomidine. *Clin Pharmacokinet* 2017;56(8):893-913.

104 Lin L, Guo X, Zhang MZ, et al. Pharmacokinetics of dexmedetomidine in Chinese post-surgical intensive care unit patients. *Acta Anaesthesiol Scand* 2011;55(3):359-67.

105 Iirola T, Ihmsen H, Laitio R, et al. Population pharmacokinetics of dexmedetomidine during long-term sedation in intensive care patients. *Br J Anaesth* 2012;108(3):460-68.

106 Cortinez LI, Anderson BJ, Holford NH, et al. Dexmedetomidine pharmacokinetics in the obese. *Eur J Clin Pharmacol* 2015;71(12):1501-08.

107 Kuang Y, Xiang YX, Guo CX, et al. Population pharmacokinetics study of dexmedetomidine in Chinese adult patients during spinal anesthesia. *Int J Clin Pharm Ther* 2016;54(3):200-07.

108 Talke P, Richardson CA, Scheinin M, et al. Postoperative pharmacokinetics and sympatholytic effects of dexmedetomidine. *Anesth Analg* 1997;85(5):1136-42.

109 Valitalo PA, Ahtola-Satila T, Wighton A, et al. Population pharmacokinetics of dexmedetomidine in critically ill patients. *Clinical drug investigation* 2013;33(8):579-87.

110 Venn RM, Karol MD, Grounds RM. Pharmacokinetics of dexmedetomidine infusions for sedation of postoperative patients requiring intensive care. *Br J Anaesth* 2002;88(5):669-75.

111 Iirola T, Aantaa R, Laitio R, et al. Pharmacokinetics of prolonged infusion of high-dose dexmedetomidine in critically ill patients. *Critical Care (London, England)* 2011;15(5):R257.

112 Lee S, Kim BH, Lim K, et al. Pharmacokinetics and pharmacodynamics of intravenous dexmedetomidine in healthy Korean subjects. *J Clin Pharm Ther* 2012;37(6):698-703.

113 Dutta S, Karol MD, Cohen T, et al. Effect of dexmedetomidine on propofol requirements in healthy subjects. *Journal of Pharmaceutical Sciences* 2001;90(2):172-81.

114 Dyck JB, Maze M, Haack C, et al. Computer-controlled infusion of intravenous dexmedetomidine hydrochloride in adult human volunteers. *Anesthesiology* 1993;78:821-28.

115 Colin PJ, Hannivoort LN, Eleveld DJ, et al. Dexmedetomidine pharmacokinetic-pharmacodynamic modelling in healthy volunteers: 1. Influence of arousal on bispectral index and sedation. *Br J Anaesth* 2017;119(2):200-10.

116 Colin PJ, Hannivoort LN, Eleveld DJ, et al. Dexmedetomidine pharmacodynamics in healthy volunteers: 2. Haemodynamic profile. *Br J Anaesth* 2017;119(2):211-20.

117 Rolle A, Paredes S, Cortinez LI, et al. Dexmedetomidine metabolic clearance is not affected by fat mass in obese patients. *Br J Anaesth* 2018;120(5):969-77.

118 Dutta S, Lal R, Karol MD, et al. Influence of cardiac output on dexmedetomidine pharmacokinetics. *Journal of Pharmaceutical Sciences* 2000;89(4):519-27.

119 Potts AL, Anderson BJ, Warman GR, et al. Dexmedetomidine pharmacokinetics in pediatric intensive care – a pooled analysis. *Paediatric anaesthesia* 2009;19(11):1119-29.

120 Wiczling P, Bartkowska-Sniatkowska A, Szerkus O, et al. The pharmacokinetics of dexmedetomidine during long-term infusion in critically ill pediatric patients. A Bayesian approach with informative priors. *J Pharmacokinet Pharmacodyn* 2016;43(3):315-24.

121 Su F, Gastonguay MR, Nicolson SC, et al. Dexmedetomidine Pharmacology in Neonates and Infants After Open Heart Surgery. *Anesth Analg* 2016;122(5):1556-66.

122 Su F, Nicolson SC, Gastonguay MR, et al. Population pharmacokinetics of dexmedetomidine in infants after open heart surgery. *Anesth Analg* 2010;110(5):1383-92.

123 Liu HC, Lian QQ, Wu FF, et al. Population Pharmacokinetics of Dexmedetomidine After Short Intravenous Infusion in Chinese Children. *Eur J Drug Metab Pharmacokinet* 2017;42(2):201-11.

124 Potts AL, Warman GR, Anderson BJ. Dexmedetomidine disposition in children: a population analysis. *Paediatr Anaesth* 2008;18(8):722-30.

125 Su X, Meng ZT, Wu XH, et al. Dexmedetomidine for prevention of delirium in elderly patients after non-cardiac surgery: a randomised, double-blind, placebo-controlled trial. *Lancet (London, England)* 2016;388(10054):1893-902.

126 White PF, Ham J, Way WL, et al. Pharmacology of ketamine isomers in surgical patients. *Anesthesiology* 1980;52(3):231-39.

127 Domino EF, Zsigmond EK, Domino LE, et al. Plasma levels of ketamine and two of its metabolites in surgical patients using a gas chromatographic mass fragmentographic assay. *Anesth Analg* 1982;61(2):87-92.

128 Domino EF, Domino SE, Smith RE, et al. Ketamine kinetics in unmedicated and diazepam-premedicated subjects. *Clin Pharmacol Ther* 1984;36(5):645-53.

129 White PF, Schuttler J, Shafer A, et al. Comparative pharmacology of the ketamine isomers. Studies in volunteers. *Br J Anaesth* 1985;57(2):197-203.

130 Geisslinger G, Hering W, Thomann P, et al. Pharmacokinetics and pharmacodynamics of ketamine enantiomers in surgical patients using a stereoselective analytical method. *Br J Anaesth* 1993;70(6):666-71.

131 Geisslinger G, Hering W, Kamp HD, et al. Pharmacokinetics of ketamine enantiomers. *Br J Anaesth* 1995;75(4):506-07.

132 Ihmsen H, Geisslinger G, Schuttler J. Stereoselective pharmacokinetics of ketamine: R(-)-ketamine inhibits the elimination of S(+)-ketamine. *Clin Pharmacol Ther* 2001;70(5):431-38.

133 White M, de Graaff P, Renshof B, et al. Pharmacokinetics of S(+) ketamine derived from target controlled infusion. *Br J Anaesth* 2006;96(3):330-34.

134 Bourgoin A, Albanese J, Leone M, et al. Effects of sufentanil or ketamine administered in target-controlled infusion on the cerebral haemodynamics of severely brain-injured patients. *Crit Care Med* 2005;33(5):1109-13.

135 Hijazi Y, Bodonian C, Bolon M, et al. Pharmacokinetics and haemodynamics of ketamine in intensive care patients with brain or spinal cord injury. *Br J Anaesth* 2003;90(2):155-60.

136 Gray C, Swinhoe CF, Myint Y, et al. Target controlled infusion of ketamine as analgesia for TIVA with propofol. *Can J Anaesth* 1999;46(10):957-61.

137 Corlett PR, Cambridge V, Gardner JM, et al. Ketamine effects on memory reconsolidation favor a learning model of delusions. *PLoS One* 2013;8(6):e65088.

138 Honey GD, Corlett PR, Absalom AR, et al. Individual differences in psychotic effects of ketamine are predicted by brain function measured under placebo. *J Neurosci* 2008;28(25):6295-303.

139 Luginbuhl M, Gerber A, Schnider TW, et al. Modulation of remifentanil-induced analgesia, hyperalgesia, and tolerance by small-dose ketamine in humans. *Anesth Analg* 2003;96(3):726-32.

140 Rogers R, Wise RG, Painter DJ, et al. An investigation to dissociate the analgesic and anesthetic properties of ketamine using functional magnetic resonance imaging. *Anesthesiology* 2004;100(2):292-301.

141 Clements JA, Nimmo WS. Pharmacokinetics and analgesic effect of ketamine in man. *Br J Anaesth* 1981;53(1):27-30.

142 Adapa RM, Axell RG, Mangat JS, et al. Safety and performance of TCI pumps in a magnetic resonance imaging environment. *Anaesthesia* 2012;67(1):33-9.

143 Varvel JR, Donoho DL, Shafer SL. Measuring the predictive performance of computer-controlled infusion pumps. *J Pharmacokinet Biopharm* 1992;20(1):63-94.

144 Schuttler J, Kloos S, Schwilden H, et al. Total intravenous anaesthesia with propofol and alfentanil by computer-assisted infusion. *Anaesthesia* 1988;43 Suppl:2-7.

145 Glass PJA, Jacobs JR, Reves JG, et al. Intravenous drug delivery. Anesthesia. New York: Churchill Livingstone 1990:367.

146 Frei FJ, Zbinden AM, Thomson DA, et al. Is the end-tidal partial pressure of isoflurane a good predictor of its arterial partial pressure? *Br J Anaesth* 1991;66(3):331-9.

147 Dwyer RC, Fee JP, Howard PJ, et al. Arterial washing of halothane and isoflurane in young and elderly adult patients. *Br J Anaesth* 1991;66(5):572-9.

148 Lee YH, Choi GH, Jung KW, et al. Predictive performance of the modified Marsh and Schnider models for propofol in underweight patients undergoing general anaesthesia using target-controlled infusion. *Br J Anaesth* 2017;118(6):883-91.

149 Rigouzzo A, Girault L, Louvet N, et al. The relationship between bispectral index and propofol during target-controlled infusion anesthesia: a comparative study between children and young adults. *Anesth Analg* 2008;106(4):1109-16.

150 Doufas AG, Bakhshandeh M, Bjorksten AR, et al. Induction speed is not a determinant of propofol pharmacodynamics. *Anesthesiology* 2004;101(5):1112-21.

151 Sahinovic MM, Eleveld DJ, Miyabe-Nishiwaki T, et al. Pharmacokinetics and pharmacodynamics of propofol: changes in patients with frontal brain tumours. *Br J Anaesth* 2017;118(6):901-09.

152 Short TG, Aun CS, Tan P, et al. A prospective evaluation of pharmacokinetic model controlled infusion of propofol in paediatric patients. *Br J Anaesth* 1994;72(3):302-06.

153 Barvais L, Heitz D, Schmartz D, et al. Pharmacokinetic model-driven infusion of sufentanil and midazolam during cardiac surgery: assessment of the prospective predictive accuracy and the quality of anesthesia. *J Cardiothorac Vasc Anesth* 2000;14(4):402-08.

154 Pandin PC, Cantraine F, Ewalenko P, et al. Predictive accuracy of target-controlled propofol and sufentanil coinfusion in long-lasting surgery. *Anesthesiology* 2000;93(3):653-61.

155 Hudson RJ, Henderson BT, Thomson IR, et al. Pharmacokinetics of sufentanil in patients undergoing coronary artery bypass graft surgery. *J Cardiothorac Vasc Anesth* 2001;15(6):693-99.

156 Slepchenko G, Simon N, Goubaux B, et al. Performance of target-controlled sufentanil infusion in obese patients. *Anesthesiology* 2003;98(1):65-73.

157 Maitre PO, Ausems ME, Vozeh S, et al. Evaluating the accuracy of using population pharmacokinetic data to predict plasma concentrations of alfentanil. *Anesthesiology* 1988;68:59-67.

158 Barvais L, d Hollander A, Schmartz D, et al. Predictive accuracy of alfentanil infusion in coronary artery surgery: a prebypass study in middle-aged and elderly patients. *JCardiothoracVascAnesth* 1994;8:278-83.

159 Absalom AR, Lee M, Menon DK, et al. Predictive performance of the Domino, Hijazi, and Clements models during low-dose target-controlled ketamine infusions in healthy volunteers. *Br J Anaesth* 2007;98(5):615-23.

160 Matot I, Neely CF, Katz RY, et al. Pulmonary uptake of propofol in cats. Effect of fentanyl and halothane. *Anesthesiology* 1993;78(6):1157-65.

161 Baker MT, Chadam MV, Ronnenberg WC, Jr. Inhibitory effects of propofol on cytochrome P450 activities in rat hepatic microsomes. *Anesth Analg* 1993;76(4):817-21.

162 Mertens MJ, Vuyk J, Olofsen E, et al. Propofol alters the pharmacokinetics of alfentanil in healthy male volunteers. *Anesthesiology* 2001;94(6):949-57.

163 Cockshott ID, Briggs LP, Douglas EJ, et al. Pharmacokinetics of propofol in female patients. Studies using single bolus injections. *British Journal of Anaesthesia* 1987;59(9):1103-10.

164 Pavlin DJ, Coda B, Shen DD, et al. Effects of combining propofol and alfentanil on ventilation, analgesia, sedation, and emesis in human volunteers. *Anesthesiology* 1996;84(1):23-37.

165 Bouillon T, Bruhn J, Radu-Radulescu L, et al. A model of the ventilatory depressant potency of remifentanil in the non-steady state. *Anesthesiology* 2003;99(4):779-87.

166 Absalom AR, Sear JW. Intravenous Anaesthetics. In: Hardman J, HopkinsP.M., M.M.R.F. S, eds. Oxford Textbook of Anaesthesia. Oxford: Oxford University Press 2017.

167 Struys MMRF, Absalom AR, Shafer SL. Intravenous drug delivery systems. In: Miller RD, Eriksson L, Fleisher A, et al., eds. Miller's Anesthesia. Philadelphia: Elsevier 2014:919-57.

168 Absalom AR, Mason KP. Total intravenous anesthesia and target controlled infusions: a comprehensive global anthology. Switzerland: Springer, 2017.

169 Leslie K, Sessler DI, Schroeder M, et al. Propofol blood concentration and the Bispectral Index predict suppression of learning during propofol/epidural anesthesia in volunteers. *Anesth Analg* 1995;81(6):1269-74.

170 Irwin MG, Thompson N, Kenny GN. Patient-maintained propofol sedation. Assessment of a target-controlled infusion system. *Anaesthesia* 1997;52(6):525-30.

171 Murdoch JA, Kenny GN. Patient-maintained propofol sedation as premedication in day-case surgery: assessment of a target-controlled system. *Br J Anaesth* 1999;82(3):429-31.

172 McMurray TJ, Johnston JR, Milligan KR, et al. Propofol sedation using Diprifusor target-controlled infusion in adult intensive care unit patients. *Anaesthesia* 2004;59(7):636-41.

173 Struys MM, Vereecke H, Moerman A, et al. Ability of the bispectral index, autoregressive modelling with exogenous input-derived auditory evoked potentials, and predicted propofol concentrations to measure patient responsiveness during anesthesia with propofol and remifentanil. *Anesthesiology* 2003;99(4):802-12.

174 LaPierre CD, Johnson KB, Randall BR, et al. An exploration of remifentanil-propofol combinations that lead to a loss of response to esophageal instrumentation, a loss of responsiveness, and/or onset of intolerable ventilatory depression. *Anesth Analg* 2011;113(3):490-99.

175 Davidson JA, Macleod AD, Howie JC, et al. Effective concentration 50 for propofol with and without 67% nitrous oxide. *Acta Anaesthesiol Scand* 1993;37:458-64.

176 Sahinovic MM, Beese U, Heeremans EH, et al. Bispectral index values and propofol concentrations at loss and return of consciousness in patients with frontal brain tumours and control patients. *Br J Anaesth* 2014;112(1):110-7.

177 Schuttler J, Stoeckel H, Schwilden H. Pharmacokinetic and pharmacodynamic modelling of propofol ('Diprivan') in volunteers and surgical patients. *Postgrad Med J* 1985;61 Suppl 3:53-54.

178 Stuart PC, Stott SM, Millar A, et al. Cp50 of propofol with and without nitrous oxide 67%. *Br J Anaesth* 2000;84(5):638-39.

179 Coppens M, Van Limmen JG, Schnider T, et al. Study of the time course of the clinical effect of propofol compared with the time course of the predicted effect-site concentration: Performance of three pharmacokinetic-dynamic models. *Br J Anaesth* 2010;104(4):452-58.

180 Bailey JM, Schwieger IM, Hug CC, Jr. Evaluation of sufentanil anesthesia obtained by a computer-controlled infusion for cardiac surgery. *Anesth Analg* 1993;76(2):247-52.

181 Ausems ME, Hug CC. Plasma concentrations of alfentanil required to supplement nitrous oxide anaesthesia for lower abdominal surgery. *Br J Anaesth* 1983;55 Suppl 2:191S-97S.

182 Ausems ME, Hug CC, Jr., Stanski DR, et al. Plasma concentrations of alfentanil required to supplement nitrous oxide anesthesia for general surgery. *Anesthesiology* 1986;65(4):362-73.

183 Vuyk J, Lim T, Engbers FH, et al. Pharmacodynamics of alfentanil as a supplement to propofol or nitrous oxide for lower abdominal surgery in female patients. *Anesthesiology* 1993;78:1036-45.

184 Smith C, McEwan AI, Jhaveri R, et al. The interaction of fentanyl on the Cp50 of propofol for loss of consciousness and skin incision. *Anesthesiology* 1994;81:820-28.

185 Kazama T, Ikeda K, Morita K. The pharmacodynamic interaction between propofol and fentanyl with respect to the suppression of somatic or haemodynamic responses to skin incision, peritoneum incision, and abdominal wall retraction. *Anesthesiology* 1998;89(4):894-906.

186 Cortinez LI, Munoz HR, De la Fuente R, et al. Target-controlled infusion of remifentanil or fentanyl during extra-corporeal shock-wave lithotripsy. *Eur J Anaesth* 2005;22(1):56-61.

187 Nagels W, Demeyere R, Van Hemelrijck J, et al. Evaluation of the neuroprotective effects of S(+)-ketamine during open-heart surgery. *Anesth Analg* 2004;98(6):1595-603.

188 Koppert W, Sittl R, Scheuber K, et al. Differential modulation of remifentanil-induced analgesia and postinfusion hyperalgesia by S-ketamine and clonidine in humans. *Anesthesiology* 2003;99(1):152-59.

189 Bell RF, Dahl JB, Moore RA, et al. Perioperative ketamine for acute postoperative pain. *Cochrane Database Syst Rev* 2006(1):CD004603.

190 Avidan MS, Maybrier HR, Abdallah AB, et al. Intraoperative ketamine for prevention of postoperative delirium or pain after major surgery in older adults: an international, multicentre, double-blind, randomised clinical trial. *Lancet (London, England)* 2017;390(10091):267-75.

191 McEwan AI, Smith C, Dyar O, et al. Isoflurane minimum alveolar concentration reduction by fentanyl. *Anesthesiology* 1993;78(5):864-69.

192 Katoh T, Kobayashi S, Suzuki A, et al. The effect of fentanyl on sevoflurane requirements for somatic and sympathetic responses to surgical incision. *Anesthesiology* 1999;90(2):398-405.

193 Westmoreland CL, Sebel PS, Gropper A. Fentanyl or alfentanil decreases the minimum alveolar anesthetic concentration of isoflurane in surgical patients. *Anesth Analg* 1994;78(1):23-8.

194 Conway DH, Hasan SK, Simpson ME. Target-controlled propofol requirements at induction of anaesthesia: effect of remifentanil and midazolam. *Eur J Anaesthesiol* 2002;19(8):580-84.

195 Cressey DM, Claydon P, Bhaskaran NC, et al. Effect of midazolam pretreatment on induction dose requirements of propofol in combination with fentanyl in younger and older adults. *Anaesthesia* 2001;56(2):108-13.

196 Rigby-Jones AE, Nolan JA, Priston MJ, et al. Pharmacokinetics of propofol infusions in critically ill neonates, infants, and children in an intensive care unit. *Anesthesiology* 2002;97(6):1393-400.

197 Richards MJ, Skues MA, Jarvis AP, et al. Total i.v. anaesthesia with propofol and alfentanil: dose requirements for propofol and the effect of premedication with clonidine. *Br J Anaesth* 1990;65(2):157-63.

198 Johansen JW, Flaishon R, Sebel PS. Esmolol reduces anesthetic requirement for skin incision during propofol/nitrous oxide/morphine anesthesia. *Anesthesiology* 1997;86(2):364-71.

199 Korpinen R, Saarnivaara L, Siren K, et al. Modification of the haemodynamic responses to induction of anaesthesia and tracheal intubation with alfentanil, esmolol and their combination. *Can J Anaesth* 1995;42(4):298-304.

200 Smith I, Van Hemelrijck J, White PF. Efficacy of esmolol versus alfentanil as a supplement to propofol-nitrous oxide anesthesia. *Anesth Analg* 1991;73(5):540-6.

201 Wilson ES, McKinlay S, Crawford JM, et al. The influence of esmolol on the dose of propofol required for induction of anaesthesia. *Anaesthesia* 2004;59(2):122-26.

202 Shafer SL, Hendrickx JF, Flood P, et al. Additivity versus synergy: a theoretical analysis of implications for anesthetic mechanisms. *Anesth Analg* 2008;107(2):507-24.

203 Eger EI, 2nd, Tang M, Liao M, et al. Inhaled anesthetics do not combine to produce synergistic effects regarding minimum alveolar anesthetic concentration in rats. *Anesth Analg* 2008;107(2):479-85.

204 Hendrickx JF, Eger EI, Sonner JM, et al. Is synergy the rule? A review of anesthetic interactions producing hypnosis and immobility. *Anesth Analg* 2008;107(2):494-506.

205 van den Berg JP, Vereecke HE, Proost JH, et al. Pharmacokinetic and pharmacodynamic interactions in anaesthesia. A review of current knowledge and how it can be used to optimize anaesthetic drug administration. *Br J Anaesth* 2017;118(1):44-57.

206 Vuyk J, Engbers FH, Burm AL, et al. Pharmacodynamic interaction between propofol and alfentanil when given for induction of anesthesia. *Anesthesiology* 1996;84(2):288-99.

207 Minto CF, Schnider TW, Short TG, et al. Response surface model for anesthetic drug interactions. *Anesthesiology* 2000;92(6):1603-16.

208 Bouillon TW, Bruhn J, Radulescu L, et al. Pharmacodynamic interaction between propofol and remifentanil regarding hypnosis, tolerance of laryngoscopy, bispectral index, and electroencephalographic approximate entropy. *Anesthesiology* 2004;100(6):1353-72.

209 Hannivoort LN, Vereecke HE, Proost JH, et al. Probability to tolerate laryngoscopy and noxious stimulation response index as general indicators of the anaesthetic potency of sevoflurane, propofol, and remifentanil. *Br J Anaesth* 2016;116(5):624-31.

210 van den Berg JP, Absalom AR, Venema AM, et al. Comparison of haemodynamic and electroencephalographic effects evoked by target-controlled infusion of propofol and remifentanil towards four equipotent conditions of tolerance to laryngoscopy. *Anesth Analg* 2019;In press

211 Nieuwenhuijs DJ, Olofsen E, Romberg RR, et al. Response surface modeling of remifentanil-propofol interaction on cardiorespiratory control and bispectral index. *Anesthesiology* 2003;98(2):312-22.

212 Weerink MAS, Barends CRM, Muskiet ERR, et al. Pharmacodynamic interaction of remifentanil and dexmedetomidine on depth of sedation and tolerance of laryngoscopy. . *Anesthesiology* 2019;In press.

213 Roberts FL, Dixon J, Lewis GT, et al. Induction and maintenance of propofol anaesthesia. A manual infusion scheme. *Anaesthesia* 1988;43 Suppl:14-17.

214 Glass P, Shafer S, Reves J. Intravenous drug delivery systems. In: Miller R, ed. Anesthesia. 5th ed. New York: Churchill-Livingstone 2000:377-411.

215 Nimmo AF, Absalom AR, Bagshaw O, et al. Guidelines for the safe practice of total intravenous anaesthesia (TIVA): Joint Guidelines from the Association of Anaesthetists and the Society for Intravenous Anaesthesia. *Anaesthesia* 2019;74(2):211-24.

216 Egan TD. Remifentanil pharmacokinetics and pharmacodynamics. A preliminary appraisal. *Clinical Pharmacokinetics* 1995;29(2):80-94.

217 Scott JC, Ponganis KV, Stanski DR. EEG quantitation of narcotic effect: the comparative pharmacodynamics of fentanyl and alfentanil. *Anesthesiology* 1985;62:234-41.

218 Scott JC, Cooke JE, Stanski DR. Electroencephalographic quantitation of opioid effect: comparative pharmacodynamics of fentanyl and sufentanil. *Anesthesiology* 1991;74:34-42.

219 Shafer SL, Varvel JR. Pharmacokinetics, pharmacodynamics, and rational opioid selection. *Anesthesiology* 1991;74(1):53-63.

220 Leslie K, Crankshaw DP. Lean tissue mass is a useful predictor of induction dose requirements for propofol. *Anaesth Intensive Care* 1991;19(1):57-60.

221 Wulfsohn NL, Joshi CW. Thiopentone dosage based on lean body ms. *Br J Anaesth* 1969;41(6):516-21.

222 Beemer GH, Bjorksten AR, Crankshaw DP. Pharmacokinetics of atracurium during continuous infusion. *Br J Anaesth* 1990;65(5):668-74.

223 Al-Sallami HS, Goulding A, Grant A, et al. Prediction of Fat-Free Mass in Children. *Clin Pharmacokinet* 2015;54(11):1169-78.

224 Abernethy DR, Greenblatt DJ, Divoll M, et al. Alterations in drug distribution and clearance due to obesity. *J Pharmacol Exp Ther* 1981;217(3):681-5.

225 Albertin A, Poli D, La Colla L, et al. Predictive performance of 'Servin's formula' during BIS-guided propofol-remifentanil target-controlled infusion in morbidly obese patients. *Br J Anaesth* 2007;98(1):66-75.

226 Cortinez LI, De la Fuente N, Eleveld DJ, et al. Performance of propofol target-controlled infusion models in the obese: pharmacokinetic and pharmacodynamic analysis. *Anesth Analg* 2014;119(2):302-10.

227 Munoz HR, Cortinez LI, Altermatt FR, et al. Remifentanil requirements during sevoflurane administration to block somatic and cardiovascular responses to skin incision in children and adults. *Anesthesiology* 2002;97(5):1142-45.

228 Thurlow JA, Laxton CH, Dick A, et al. Remifentanil by patient-controlled analgesia compared with intramuscular meperidine for pain relief in labour. *Br J Anaesth* 2002;88(3):374-78.

229 McCarroll CP, Paxton LD, Elliott P, et al. Use of remifentanil in a patient with peripartum cardiomyopathy requiring Caesarean section. *Br J Anaesth* 2001;86(1):135-38.

230 Blair JM, Hill DA, Fee JP. Patient-controlled analgesia for labour using remifentanil: a feasibility study. *Br J Anaesth* 2001;87(3):415-20.

231 Gallagher G, Rae CP, Kenny GN, et al. The use of a target-controlled infusion of alfentanil to provide analgesia for burn dressing changes. A dose finding study. *Anaesthesia* 2000;55(12):1159-63.

232 Irwin MG, Jones RD, Visram AR, et al. Patient-controlled alfentanil. Target-controlled infusion for postoperative analgesia. *Anaesthesia* 1996;51(5):427-30.

233 Turfrey DJ, Ray DA, Sutcliffe NP, et al. Thoracic epidural anaesthesia for coronary artery bypass graft surgery. Effects on postoperative complications. *Anaesthesia* 1997;52(11):1090-5.

234 Checketts MR, Gilhooly CJ, Kenny GN. Patient-maintained analgesia with target-controlled alfentanil infusion after cardiac surgery: a comparison with morphine PCA. *Br J Anaesth* 1998;80(6):748-51.

235 Schraag S, Kenny GN, Mohl U, et al. Patient-maintained remifentanil target-controlled infusion for the transition to early postoperative analgesia. *Br J Anaesth* 1998;81(3):365-68.

236 Stewart JT, Warren FW, Maddox FC, et al. The stability of remifentanil hydrochloride and propofol mixtures in polypropylene syringes and polyvinylchloride bags at 22 degrees-24 degrees C. *Anesth Analg* 2000;90(6):1450-1.

237 O'Connor S, Zhang YL, Christians U, et al. Remifentanil and propofol undergo separation and layering when mixed in the same syringe for total intravenous anesthesia. *Pediatr Anesth* 2016;26(7):703-09.

238 Struys M, Valk BI, Eleveld DJ, et al. A Phase 1, Single-center, Double-blind, Placebo-controlled Study in Healthy Subjects to Assess the Safety, Tolerability, Clinical Effects, and Pharmacokinetics-Pharmacodynamics of Intravenous Cyclopropyl-methoxycarbonylmetomidate (ABP-700) after a Single Ascending Bolus Dose. *Anesthesiology* 2017;127(1):20-35.

239 Valk BI, Absalom AR, Meyer P, et al. Safety and clinical effect of i.v. infusion of cyclopropyl-methoxycarbonyl etomidate (ABP-700), a soft analogue of etomidate, in healthy subjects. *Br J Anaesth* 2018;120(6):1401-11.

240 Pastis NJ, Yarmus LB, Schippers F, et al. Safety and Efficacy of Remimazolam Compared With Placebo and Midazolam for Moderate Sedation During Bronchoscopy. *Chest* 2019;155(1):137-46.

241 Barends CRM, Absalom AR, Struys M. Drug selection for ambulatory procedural sedation. *Curr Opin Anaesthesiol* 2018;31(6):673-78.

242 Albertin A, Casati A, Bergonzi P, et al. Effects of two target-controlled concentrations (1 and 3 ng/ml) of remifentanil on MAC(BAR) of sevoflurane. *Anesthesiology* 2004;100(2):255-59.

243 Colin PJ, Jonckheere S, Struys M. Target-Controlled Continuous Infusion for Antibiotic Dosing: Proof-of-Principle in an In-silico Vancomycin Trial in Intensive Care Unit Patients. *Clin Pharmacokinet* 2018;57(11):1435-47.

244 Pasin L, Nardelli P, Pintaudi M, et al. Closed-Loop Delivery Systems Versus Manually Controlled Administration of Total IV Anesthesia: A Meta-analysis of Randomized Clinical Trials. *Anesth Analg* 2017;124(2):456-64.

245 Brogi E, Cyr S, Kazan R, et al. Clinical Performance and Safety of Closed-Loop Systems: A Systematic Review and Meta-analysis of Randomized Controlled Trials. *Anesth Analg* 2017;124(2):446-55.

246 Loeb RG, Cannesson M. Closed-Loop Anesthesia: Ready for Prime Time? *Anesth Analg* 2017;124(2):381-82.

247 Cowley NJ, Hutton P, Clutton-Brock TH. Assessment of the performance of the Marsh model in effect site mode for target controlled infusion of propofol during the maintenance phase of general anaesthesia in an unselected population of neurosurgical patients. *Eur J Anaesth* 2013;30(10):627-32.

248 Grossherr M, Hengstenberg A, Dibbelt L, et al. Blood gas partition coefficient and pulmonary extraction ratio for propofol in goats and pigs. *Xenobiotica* 2009;39(10):782-87.

249 Hornuss C, Praun S, Villinger J, et al. Real-time monitoring of propofol in expired air in humans undergoing total intravenous anesthesia. *Anesthesiology* 2007;106(4):665-74.

250 Ziaian D, Kleiboemer K, Hengstenberg A, et al. Pharmacokinetic modeling of the transition of propofol from blood plasma to breathing gas. IEEE international symposium on medical measurements and applications (MeMeA)2014:1-5.

251 Panchatsharam S, Callaghan M, Day R, et al. Measured versus predicted blood propofol concentrations in children during scoliosis surgery. *Anesth Analg* 2014;119(5):1150-57.

252 van den Berg JP, Eleveld DJ, De Smet T, et al. Influence of Bayesian optimization on the performance of propofol target-controlled infusion. *Br J Anaesth* 2017;119(5):918-27.

APPENDIX

Description of the pharmacokinetic-dynamic models

Sufentanil: Gepts model (Gepts et al. Anesthesiology 1995;83:1194-1204)

$V_1 = 14.3L$

$k_{10} = 0.0645/min$

$k_{12} = 0.1086/min$

$k_{13} = 0.0229/min$

$k_{21} = 0.0245/min$

$k_{31} = 0.0013/min$

k_{41} determined by $t_{peak} = 5.6min$ (Shafer et al. Anesthesiology 1991;74:53-63)

Propofol: Marsh model (Marsh et al. BJA 1991;67:41-48)

$Vc = 0.228 * weight (L*kg)$

$k_{10} = 0.119/min$

$k_{12} = 0.112/min$

$k_{13} = 0.0419/min$

$k_{21} = 0.055/min$

$k_{31} = 0.0033/min$

$k_{41} = 0.26/min$

Propofol: Schnider model (Schnider et al. Anesthesiology 1998:88:1170-1182)

$V_1 = 4.27 L$

$V_2 = 18.9 L - 0.391*(age-53)$

$V_3 = 238 L$

$Cl_1 = 1.89 + 0.0456*(weight-77) - 0.0681*(lbm-59) + 0.0264*(height-177)$

$Cl_2 = 1.29 - 0.024*(age-53)$

$Cl_3 = 0.836$

k_{41} determined by $t_{peak} = 1.6min$ (Schnider et al. Anesthesiology 1999;90:1502-16)

Propofol: Kataria model (Kataria et al. Anesthesiology 1994; 80:104-122)

$V_1 = 0.41*$weight

$V_2 = 0.78*$weight $+ 3.1*$age $- 16$

$V_3 = 6.9*$weight

$Cl_1 = 0.035*$weight

$Cl_2 = 0.077*$weight

$Cl_3 = 0.026*$weight

No effect-site data available

Propofol: Paedfusor model (Absalom et al. BJA 2003;91:507-513 and BJA 2005;95:110)

$V_1 =$ age 1-12: $0.4584*$weight

age = 13: $0.400*$ weight

age = 14: $0.342*$ weight

age = 15: $0.284*$ weight

age = 16: $0.228*$ weight

$k_{10} =$ age 1-12: $0.1527*($ weight $**(-0.3))$

age = 13: 0.0678

age = 14: 0.0792

age = 15: 0.0954

age >= 16: 0.119

$k_{12} = 0.114$

$k_{21} = 0.055$

$k_{13} = 0.0419$

$k_{31} = 0.0033$

Propofol: Eleveld PK-PD model (Eleveld et al. Br J Anaesth 2018;120:942-959)

FFM(weight, height, sex) = Al-Sallami equation (Al-Sallami HS, Goulding A, Grant A, Taylor R, Holford N, Duffull SB. Prediction of fat-free mass in children. Clin Pharmacokin 2015;54:1169-78)

Subscript ref are calculated for a 70 kg, 35 year, 170 cm, male, full term (40 weeks)

Fsize = weight / 70

Fage(x) = exp(-x*(age - 35))

Fsigmoid(x, e50, gamma) = x**gamma / (x**gamma + e50**gamma)

Fcentral = Fsigmoid(weight, 33.6, 1)

Fopiates(x) = absence: 1, presence: exp(x*age)

Fmatcl = Fsigmoid(post-menstrual age, 42.3 weeks, 9.06)

Fsexcl = male: 1.79, female: 2.10

Fmatq3 = Fsigmoid(age + 40 weeks, 68.3 weeks, 1)

$V_1 = 6.28*(Fcentral(weight) / Fcentral_{ref})$

$V_2 = 25.5*Fsize*Fage(-0.0156)$

$V_3 = 273*(FFM / FFMref)*Fopiates(-0.0138)$

$Cl_1 = Fsexcl*Fsize**0.75*(Fmatcl / Fmatcl_{ref})*Fopiates(-0.00286)$

$Cl_2 = 1.75*(V_2 / V_2ref)**0.75*(1 + 1.3*(1 - Fmatq3))$

$Cl_3 = 1.11*(V_3 / V_3ref)**0.75*(Fmatq3 / Fmatq3_{ref})$

$keo = 0.146*Fsize**-0.25$

$E_{50} = 3.08*Fage(-0.00635)$

Remifentanil: Minto model (Minto et al. Anesthesiology 1997;86:10-23)

LBM = male: $1.10*weight - 128*(weight/height)**2$,

female: $1.17*weight - 148*(weight/height)**2$

A = (age – 40) L = (LBM – 55)

$V_1 = 5.1 - 0.0201*A + 0.072 *L$

$V_2 = 9.82 - 0.0811*A + 0.108*L$

$V_3 = 5.42$

$Cl_1 = 2.6 - 0.0162*A + 0.0191*L$

$Cl_2 = 2.05 - 0.0301*A$

$Cl_3 = 0.076-0.00113*A$

$k_{41} = 0.595-0.007*A$

Remifentanil Eleveld (Eleveld et al. Anesthesiology 2017;126:1005-1018)

FFM(weight, height, sex) = Al-Sallami equation (Al-Sallami HS, Goulding A, Grant A, Taylor R, Holford N, Duffull SB. Prediction of fat-free mass in children. Clinical pharmacokinetics. 2015 Nov 1;54(11):1169-78.)

Subscript ref are calculated for a 70 kg, 35 year, 170 cm, male

$Fsize = FFM(weight, height, sex) / FFM_{ref}$

$Fage(x) = exp(-x*(age - 35))$

$Fsigmoid(x, e_{50}, gamma) = x**gamma / (x**gamma + e_{50}**gamma)$

Fmat(weight) = Fsigmoid(weight, 2.88, 2)

Fsex = male: 1, female: 1 + 0.47*Fsigmoid(age, 12, 6)*(1 – Fsigmoid(age, 45, 6))

$V_1 = 5.81*Fsize*Fage(-0.00554)$

$V_2 = 8.82*Fsize*Fage(-0.00327)*Fsex$

$V_3 = 5.03*Fsize*Fage(-0.0315)*exp(-0.0260*(weight - 70))$

$Cl_1 = 2.58*Fsize**0.75*(Fmat / Fmat_{ref})*Fsex*Fage(-0.00327)$

$Cl_2 = 1.72*(V_2/8.82)**0.75*Fage(-0.00554)*Fsex$

$Cl_3 = 0.124*(V_3/5.03)**0.75*Fage(-0.00554)$

$keo = 1.09*Fage(-0.0289)$

Remifentanil: Kim model (Kim et al. Anesthesiology 2017 ;126 :1019-103)
FFM(weight, height, sex)=Janmahasatian (Janmahasatian S, Duffull SB, Ash S, Ward LC, Byrne NM, Green B. Quantification of lean bodyweight. Clinical pharmacokinetics. 2005, 44, 1051-65)

$V_1 = 4.76^*(\text{weight} / 74.5)^{**}0.658$

$V_2 = 8.4^*(\text{FFM} / 52.3)^{**}0.573 - 0.0936^*(\text{age} - 37)$

$V_3 = 4 - 0.0477^*(\text{age} - 37)$

$Cl_1 = 2.77^*(\text{weight} / 74.5)^{**}0.336 - 0.0149^*(\text{age} - 37)$

$Cl_2 = 1.94 - 0.0280^*(\text{age} - 37)$

$Cl_3 = 0.197$

Alfentanil: Maitre model (Maitre et al. Anesthesiology 1987 ;66:3-12)

V_1 = male: 0.111^*weight, female: $0.111^*1.15^*$ weight

Cl_1 = Age <= 40: 0.356, else $0.356 - 0.00269^*(\text{age} - 40)$

$k_{10} = Cl_1/V_1$

$k_{12} = 0.104$

$k_{13} = 0.017$

$k_{21} = 0.0673$

k_{31} = Age <= 40: 0.0126, else $0.0126 - 0.000113^*(\text{age} - 40)$

k_{41} determined by t_{peak} = 1.4min (Shafer, Anesthesiology 1991, 74, 53-63)

Dexmedetomidine: Hannivoort – Colin model (Hannivoort et al. Anesthesiology 2015;123:357-67 ; Colin et al. BJA 2017 ;119:200-210 ; Colin et al. BJA. 2017;119:211-220)

$V_1 = 1.78^*(\text{weight} / 70)$

$V_2 = 30.3^*(\text{weight} / 70)$

$V_3 = 52.0^*(\text{weight} / 70)$

$Cl_1 = 0.686^*(\text{weight} / 70)^{**}0.75$

$Cl_2 = 2.98^*(V_2 / 30.3)^{**}0.75$

$Cl_3 = 0.602^*(V_3 / 52.0)^{**}0.75$

$keo(\text{BIS}) = 0.120$

$keo(\text{MOAA/S}) = 0.04$ 28

$keo(\text{MAP, hypo}) = 0.0529$

$keo(\text{MAP, hyper}) = 0.0902$

$keo(\text{HR}) = 0.396$